To my patients and to Helle, Eva, and Niels

THE
HEART ATTACK
HANDBOOK

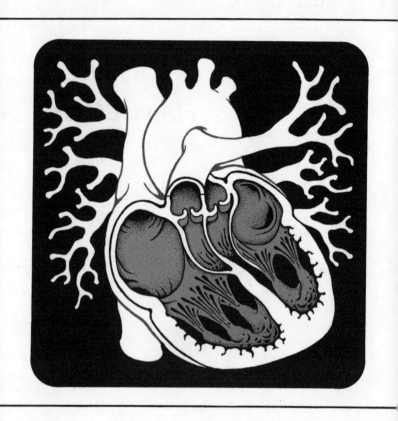

THE HEART ATTACK HANDBOOK

A Commonsense Guide to Treatment, Recovery, and Staying Well

by Joseph S. Alpert, M.D.

Little, Brown and Company
Boston / Toronto

Third Printing

LIBRARY OF CONGRESS CATALOGING IN PUBLICATION DATA

Alpert, Joseph S
  The heart attack handbook.

  Bibliography: p.
  1. Heart—Infarction. I. Title.
[DNLM: 1. Coronary disease—Popular works. WG113
A456h]
RC685.I6A45 616.1'23 78-1978
ISBN 0-316-03501-7

Illustrations by Jim Chiros.

Figures 8 and 9 from *Understanding Human Sexual Inadequacy* by Fred Belliveau and Lin Richter. Copyright © 1970 by Fred Belliveau and Lin Richter. Reprinted by permission of Little, Brown and Company.

Designed by Janis Capone

Published simultaneously in Canada
by Little, Brown & Company (Canada) Limited

PRINTED IN THE UNITED STATES OF AMERICA

CONTENTS

One morning at breakfast, my wife suggested that I write this book. During the succeeding weeks, I discussed the idea with a number of my patients. All of them felt the need for a concise, understandable guide to the causes and remedies of a heart attack. This book was written to answer the many questions and to quiet the myriad anxieties that arise following a myocardial infarction, or heart attack. It is my hope that reading this book will help to fill some of the many boring hours while the patient is recovering in the hospital or at home. Although I have tried to sketch an average cardiologist's program for recovery from a heart attack, there will be a number of differences between the advice in this book and that of the thousands of American physicians caring for heart attack patients. Needless to say, many different routes lead to the same goal, and this brief handbook should certainly not be interpreted as a policy statement of what constitutes appropriate medical care following myocardial infarction. Rather, this guide is intended to supplement the advice of the patient's own physician.

I would like to acknowledge the inspiration and assistance of the following individuals (alphabetically arranged) : Mrs. Jane Alexander, R.N., M.S.N., Cardiac Clinical Nurse, Peter Bent Brigham Hospital; Dr. Eugene Braunwald, Chief of Medicine, Peter Bent Brigham Hospital; Dr. Gary S. Francis, Director of the Coronary Care Unit, Hennepin County General Hospital, Minneapolis; Dr. Howard Horn, Cardiologist, Peter Bent Brigham Hospital; Dr. Kenneth Shine, Chief of the Cardiology Division, U.C.L.A. Medical Center, Los Angeles; and Dr. Thomas W. Smith, Chief of the Cardiovascular Division, Peter Bent Brigham Hospital.

I would also like to express my gratitude to Mrs. Gertrude Campbell, Chief Nurse, Coronary Care Unit, Naval Regional Medical Center, San Diego, and Mrs. Barbara MacDonald, Chief Nurse, Levine Cardiac Unit, Peter Bent Brigham Hospital, both of whom have taught me a great deal about heart attack patients. I would also like to thank my secretary, Mrs. Susan Hanson, as well as Lin Richter and Win Hodges of Little, Brown and Company for help in all phases of the preparation of this book.
J. S. A.

THE
HEART ATTACK
HANDBOOK

You — or someone you know — may have recently suffered a heart attack, or, as the medical profession calls it, a myocardial infarction. In medical terminology, *myo* means muscle and *cardial* refers to the heart. Infarction is a process by which part of an organ dies because of cessation of blood flow to that organ. Thus, a myocardial infarction is the death of a piece of heart muscle because of a decrease in the flow of blood to the heart muscle itself. Medical personnel frequently use the abbreviation MI for myocardial infarction.

Having a heart attack can be a frightening experience. Some patients react to a heart attack by being just plain scared. Others ignore the problem, out of fear, and deny that anything is amiss. Both of these responses are quite normal, but they can interfere with the treatment program and render it less effective. Learning about the process that leads to myocardial infarction and the methods used to treat it helps to reduce fear and denial. The relief of fear and denial through learning is what this book is about. It explains how the heart functions, what went wrong when the heart attack occurred, and which route to recovery is best.

Many patients believe that a heart attack is a definite sign their life is about to end. Others expect to lead the life of a semi-invalid after discharge from the hospital. Nothing could be farther from the truth! Remember that Presidents Eisenhower and Johnson suffered a number of heart attacks before, during, and after their terms in the White House. Despite their heart attacks, they both continued full and vigorous lives, performing the duties of the most stressful job in the world. Every community in the United States has examples of people like Presidents Eisenhower and Johnson: individuals who lead active and productive lives despite previous heart attacks.

Every person is unique, and every doctor has his/her own style and method of treating heart attack patients. But certain elements in the treatment of myocardial infarction are the same for all doctors and hospitals. Such elements include reduced activity for a variable period of time after the attack and suggested changes in life-style for the patient after his/her discharge from the hospital. These changes include stopping cigarette smoking, losing weight, and decreasing physical and psychological stress. Other specific changes may include medication to regulate the heart, blood pressure, or blood cholesterol level, and a graded exercise program. This book explains the cause and effect of a heart attack and the various therapies employed in the treatment of myocardial infarction.

There are also a glossary and appendices containing a list of medications commonly prescribed for patients who have had heart attacks.

Part 1.
THE HEART ATTACK

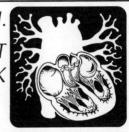

1.
How the Heart and Circulatory System Work

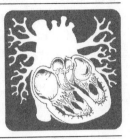

The heart is a muscle that pumps blood throughout the body (Figure 1). It is divided into a right side, pumping blood to the lungs, and a left side, pumping blood to the rest of the body. Each of the two sides of the heart contains a pumping chamber, or ventricle, and a priming chamber, or atrium. Priming means filling up completely with fluid for efficient pumping. The atrium completely fills the ventricle by squeezing its blood into the ventricle before the latter begins its pumping cycle. There are three sequential steps to a single cycle of the heart pump: 1) the atrium and ventricle fill with blood, 2) the atrium maximally fills the ventricle, and 3) the ventricle pumps blood out of the heart. In addition, the heart has four valves to ensure that the passage of blood through the heart always goes in the same direction. The valves are situated within the heart between each atrium and ventricle and between the ventricles and the main blood vessels leaving the heart. The heart is surrounded by a tough, protective membrane known as the pericardium (*peri* means around the; *cardium* means heart).

Blood is pumped by the right ventricle to the lungs in order to pick up oxygen, an essential element for life. Once the blood is fully loaded with oxygen, it returns to the left side of the heart. From here, the blood with its supply of oxygen and important nutrients is pumped throughout the body, being carried to all parts of the body through elastic, muscular tubes known as arteries. After it has nourished the various tissues of the body, blood returns to the right side of the heart via large vessels known as veins. The left ventricle is responsible for pumping the blood through the entire body and eventually back to the right atrium. Once returned to the right side of the heart, the blood is again pumped to the lungs to become refurnished with oxygen and so prepared for another circulatory journey through the rest of the body. Figure 1 demonstrates this continuous cycle. Approximately ten to fifteen seconds are required for blood to make a complete circuit in the cardiovascu-

FIGURE 1. Circulation of Blood Through the Heart

Arrows demonstrate the pathway taken by the blood as it is pumped by the right and left sides of the heart. Dark blood, low in oxygen and nutrients and high in waste products, returns to the heart via systemic veins. The blood passes into one of the two priming chambers of the heart, the right atrium. From there, the pumping chamber of the right side of the heart, the right ventricle, pumps the blood through the pulmonary artery, which divides into many branches carrying blood to all parts of the lungs. Within the lungs, blood becomes filled with oxygen and its color lightens to a bright red. This oxygenated blood returns to the left atrium via the pulmonary veins. From the left atrium the blood passes into the left ventricle, which pumps the blood into the aorta.

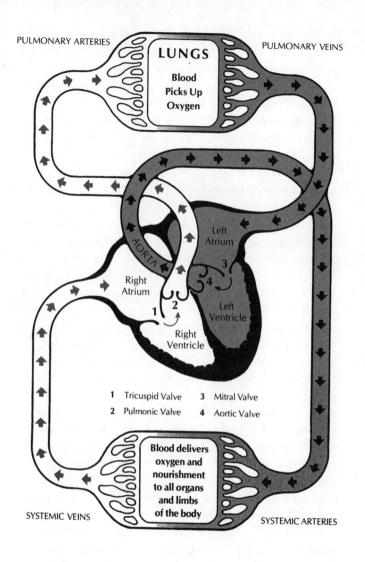

lar (heart and blood vessel) system. During a single passage of the blood through the circulatory system of a person at rest, the heart beats ten to twenty times.

The heart, like other organs in the body, must receive constant nourishment if it is to continue its vigorous pumping action. This nourishment is supplied to the heart by blood carried into it by branches of the two coronary — meaning heart — arteries. Each one of these coronary arteries supplies blood to a part of the heart muscle through numerous branches. Figure 2 shows the two coronary arteries and their branches.

All forms of muscular activity, such as walking and running, as well as digestion of meals, healing of wounds or infections, and numerous other functions, require the heart to increase the amount of blood that it pumps. Increased pumping work by the heart means an increased need in the heart muscle itself for nourishing blood. In individuals who have normal hearts and normal coronary arteries, increased pumping by the heart causes the coronary arteries to enlarge in diameter and thus deliver a larger quantity of blood to the heart muscle.

Certain disease states can narrow the coronary arteries, however, and prevent the heart from obtaining the increased amount of blood needed for various demands. Like a motor fed too little fuel, the heart supplied with too little blood functions poorly. If the amount of blood fed to the heart increases, then the pumping function of the heart will return to normal.

The heart has an intricate electrical system that enables it to beat in a coordinated and regular fashion. The electrical activity of this system is recorded on the

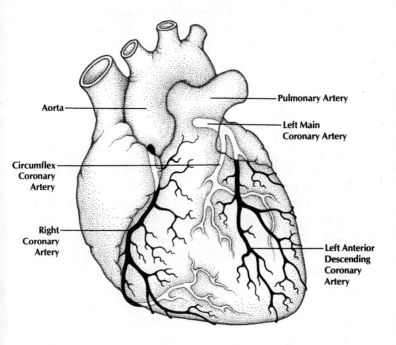

Aorta

Pulmonary Artery

Left Main
Coronary Artery

Circumflex
Coronary
Artery

Right
Coronary
Artery

Left Anterior
Descending
Coronary
Artery

This is a diagram of the main blood vessels that supply nourishing blood to the heart muscle. In this view, the segments of these blood vessels shown in black are directly visible on the surface of the heart; the parts shown in white are obscured behind other heart structures. These blood vessels have numerous branches, but the four most important ones are identified. The heart has two major coronary arteries branching off the aorta: the right coronary artery and the left main coronary artery. The left main coronary artery is short and soon divides into two major branches — the left anterior descending coronary artery and the circumflex coronary artery. The aorta and pulmonary artery are also shown.

7 / *How the Heart and Circulatory System Work*

electrocardiogram (*electro* means electrical; *cardio* means heart; *gram* means writing) , or EKG. Nerves from the brain govern the heart's electrical system so that the brain can actually speed or slow the number of times that the heart beats in a minute, the so-called heart rate. For example, if a person becomes frightened, the brain prepares the body to fight or run away. This preparation includes a sudden increase in heart rate. The analogy here is to the racing-car driver who "revs" up his motor just prior to the start of a race. Many other factors can also influence the heart rate. In healthy adults at rest, the heart beats between sixty and a hundred times per minute.

The healthy heart also maintains a certain level of blood pressure throughout the body by a combination of regulating factors: the vigor with which the left ventricle pumps the blood, the size and number of blood vessels that receive the blood from the heart, and an intricate series of checks and balances that helps control the extent to which the blood vessels are open or closed. The kidneys receive 25 percent of the blood pumped from the heart each minute, playing an important role in controlling blood pressure and the amount of fluid retained in the body. The level of the blood pressure does not depend on the heart rate. A person may have a normal heart rate and have normal, high, or low blood pressure. It is normal for blood pressure to increase briefly during exercise or emotional stress.

Blood pressure is measured at two points during the beating of the heart: when the heart is in the midst of actually pumping blood and when it is resting and filling up with blood for the next pumping cycle. The first, or pumping, phase is referred to as systole (contraction) and the second, or filling, phase is called diastole (expansion). Blood pressure is measured in millimeters of mercury, just as air pressure in automobile tires is measured in pounds per square inch. Systolic, or pumping-phase, pressure normally ranges from 100 to 140 millimeters of mercury. Diastolic, or resting phase, pressure is usually in the range of 60 to 90 millimeters of mercury. Both systolic and diastolic blood pressure can become elevated. In the shorthand of the hospital, the blood pressure is written with the systolic value over the diastolic value. For example, someone with a systolic pressure of 120 millimeters of mercury and a diastolic pressure of 80 millimeters of mercury would have his/her blood pressure written as 120/80.

Many individuals in the United States experience abnormally elevated blood pressure for long periods of time. This abnormality is known as hypertension (*hyper* means increased; *tension* means pressure). Both systolic and diastolic pressures become elevated; but raised diastolic is more serious than raised systolic pressure. The causes of this disease are incompletely understood. It appears that persons who have it are born with an abnormal blood-pressure-control mechanism, having an elevated rather than a normal setting in that part of the brain that controls blood pressure. To maintain an elevated pressure, the heart must work harder. Hypertension may also cause damage to the coronary arteries by placing undue stress on the walls of these blood vessels. Patients with hearts weakened from any of many forms of heart disease may have a difficult time pumping enough blood to maintain the pressure at a normal level.

Damage to one or more of the heart valves can result in backward movement of blood within the heart. Physicians call this valvular regurgitation. Such a defect is clearly not beneficial because the heart loses efficiency and must work overtime to make up for any blood that is pumped in the wrong direction.

2.
What Causes Heart Attacks?

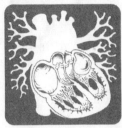

The primary cause of heart attacks is atherosclerosis, or "hardening of the arteries." In this disease process, fatty deposits such as cholesterol build up on the inside wall of the coronary arteries. This gradual process narrows the inner diameter of the coronary arteries, which in turn, cannot supply the required amount of blood to the working heart muscle. As we noted earlier, when the heart muscle cannot obtain the amount of blood that it needs to function normally, it acts like a motor whose fuel line has become clogged, that is, it operates poorly. The deposit of fatty substances such as cholesterol on the inside of the coronary arteries begins very early in life. This is a normal aging process that occurs in everyone. This aging process becomes abnormal, however, when it occurs at speeded rates. There are usually no symptoms until the narrowing is quite far advanced and very severe, and this normally would take many years. The process of atherosclerosis is very much like the corrosion and buildup of mineral deposits that take place on the inside of a pipe or plumbing system. (See Figure 3.) In

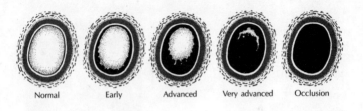

| Normal | Early | Advanced | Very advanced | Occlusion |

FIGURE 3. Stages in the Development of Atherosclerotic Narrowing of a Coronary Artery

These cross-sectional diagrams show various stages of the process by which atherosclerotic deposits narrow and eventually occlude (completely close off) a coronary artery.

addition to the heart, the brain, kidneys, and intestines can suffer serious damage when atherosclerosis narrows the arteries that supply blood to these organs.

What causes these fatty deposits to build up on the inside of the coronary arteries? No one knows for sure all of the different factors that cause atherosclerosis. A number of different causes have been identified that seem to be important: 1) **Age** — Aging is an important factor in the development of hardening of the arteries. The longer one lives and the more one's heart and blood vessels work, the greater is the chance of developing "hardening of the arteries," or atherosclerosis. 2) **Cigarette Smoking** — Cigarette smoking has been shown to damage the inner lining of the coronary arteries. This damage speeds the development of atherosclerosis. In addition, cigarette smoking hinders the blood's ability to carry life-giving oxygen. These two factors together, namely an increased propensity to develop atherosclerosis and a decreased ability of the blood to carry oxygen, strongly predispose individuals who smoke toward the development of heart attacks. **3) High Blood Pressure —** As we noted earlier, high blood pressure is extremely common in the American population. Elevated blood pressure speeds the development of atherosclerosis in the coronary arteries by damaging the inner lining of the arteries. It has been suggested that increased blood pressure "wears out" the coronary arteries faster than if a normal blood pressure had been present. **4) Elevated Cholesterol and Triglyceride Levels in the Blood —** Cholesterol and triglyceride are fatty substances that are normally present in the bloodstream. They are important fuel sources that are burned by many of the cells of the body. Some individuals have very high levels of one or both of these fat substances in their blood. Elevated cholesterol and/or triglyceride levels in the blood speed the process of atherosclerosis in the coronary arteries. In some persons, elevated cholesterol and triglyceride occur because of inherited predisposition. In others, these fatty substances increase in the bloodstream because of a diet excessively rich in saturated fat and cholesterol. **5) Inactivity —** Lack of regular exercise *may* also be a factor in hastening the development of coronary atherosclerosis. Regular exercise *may* help to increase the number and size of "reserve" blood vessels (collateral vessels) in the heart. These reserve blood vessels can take over the function of supplying the heart with blood should the original coronary arteries become blocked. Regular exercise *may* also help to decrease the buildup of atherosclerotic deposits in the coronary arteries by decreasing the level of cholesterol in the blood. **6) Obesity —** Many authorities believe that being abnormally overweight increases one's risk of developing atherosclerosis of the coronary arteries. Mild obesity is probably not a factor predisposing to the development of "hardening of the arteries," but an increase of 20 to 30 percent over one's ideal body weight may well increase one's risk of developing coronary artery narrowing. 7) **Stress** — A number of studies have suggested that increased psychological stress predisposes individuals to coronary atherosclerosis. Two personality types, called Type A and Type B, have been defined in the American population. Individuals with Type A personality are extremely time conscious. They are very compulsive about their work and are constantly concerned about "not wasting a moment." Type B personalities are more relaxed, more easygoing and less compulsive. It has been suggested that individuals with Type A personalities have a greater risk of developing "hardening of the arteries" and heart trouble. 8) **Heredity** — Certain families seem to have a propensity for developing coronary artery disease at a young age. Men are more disposed to develop coronary artery disease than are women. 9) **Diabetes** — Diabetes is an inherited disease in which the body cannot cope adequately with ingested sugars and starches (carbohydrates). This disease increases the rate at which atherosclerosis develops. It should also be noted that coffee, tea, and alcoholic beverages have *not* been shown to increase one's risk of coronary artery disease.

When the process of atherosclerosis has narrowed the passageway of the coronary arteries to a severe degree, little if any blood can get through to supply certain parts of the heart muscle. When this happens, reserve (collateral) coronary blood vessels attempt to compensate for the deficiency of blood supply to the heart. Sometimes, these reserve blood vessels provide sufficient amounts of blood to the heart so that no symptoms of heart disease arise despite quite severe narrowings of the coronary arteries. Usually, however, severe narrowings result in either the symptom of angina pectoris (see Chapter 4) or a heart attack. Sometimes a blood clot forms in an area of severe narrowing. This clot completely blocks the coronary artery and frequently a heart attack results. Blockage of a coronary artery by a blood clot is called thrombosis of the artery (from *thrombus,* meaning clot) .

Myocardial infarction can occur in one of two ways. First, as mentioned already, a coronary artery that has previously been only partially blocked by atherosclerosis may actually become totally blocked by a blood clot. When this happens, there can be a complete cessation of blood flow into part of the heart muscle, which then dies. Second, a myocardial infarction can occur when an individual with narrowings in the coronary arteries continues to exert himself despite the warning symptom of angina pectoris and continues to demand a great deal of work from the heart at a time when the heart is telling the person to slow down or cease activity. Under this stress, heart cells may actually become so deprived of nourishing blood that they die.

A myocardial infarction, or heart attack, actually entails the death or damage of a piece of the heart muscle (Figure 4) . Unlike the skin or the blood, heart muscle cannot renew itself when it dies. A scar forms in its place and the person must live on with less heart muscle available. The complete healing process takes approximately six weeks.

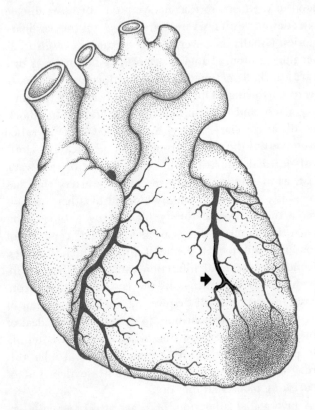

FIGURE 4. Myocardial Infarction Due to Severe Narrowing of the Anterior Descending Artery

The shaded area (lower right) depicts a myocardial infarction, or heart attack. The infarcted part of the heart has died because of the severe narrowing present in the anterior descending coronary artery (arrow).

THE HEART ATTACK / 16

In summary, then, a heart attack is the end of a long and gradual disease process, beginning early in life. The gradual buildup of fatty deposits known as atherosclerosis increasingly narrows the coronary arteries, thereby decreasing the amount of blood flow into the heart muscle. At a certain point, too little blood gets through the narrowed coronary artery and part of the heart muscle then dies. This death of a piece of heart muscle causes the symptoms of a myocardial infarction, or heart attack.

Prevention of Coronary Artery Disease

Although one cannot change inherited predispositions, age, or sex, many habits that predispose Americans to coronary artery disease can be altered (Table 1). Stopping or not starting cigarette smoking is an important measure in the prevention of coronary disease. It is also reasonable to have one's blood pressure and serum cholesterol checked each year or two. Avoiding foods rich in saturated fat and cholesterol and maintaining ideal body weight (see Chapter 9) may retard development of atherosclerosis. Regular exercise is beneficial to the heart, the lungs, and the blood vessels of the body. In addition, one should attempt to accept life as it occurs, trying to avoid the feeling of being trapped or forced to run on a never-ending treadmill. Following a life-style similar to that just described should decrease a person's chance of developing coronary artery disease. Childhood is not too early to begin checking for risk factors and eliminating them.

TABLE 1. Factors Related to the Development of Coronary Artery Disease

---

Controllable factors related to the development of coronary artery disease

Cigarette smoking
Diet rich in saturated fat and cholesterol
Elevated blood levels of cholesterol or triglyceride (hyperlipidemia)
High blood pressure (hypertension)
Diabetes
Obesity
Stress

Uncontrollable factors related to the development of coronary artery disease

Age
Heredity
Male sex
Post-menopausal state

3.
What Effect Does a Heart Attack Have on the Heart?

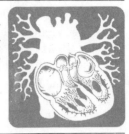

Despite the fact that a piece of heart muscle has died during the process of a heart attack, the heart must continue working. Since one cannot recover the use of heart muscle that has died, the heart must continue its work with fewer muscle cells than it had before the heart attack. Therefore each surviving heart cell must work harder. It takes a while for the surviving heart cells to accommodate themselves to their new work load. This means that the first few weeks following a heart attack are a time of particular stress for the heart, and the patient may perceive this as unusual fatigue. For this reason doctors usually recommend rest and decreased activity during the first few weeks after a heart attack. Occasionally, the insult to the heart causes it to function poorly. When the heart functions poorly, blood has a tendency to "back up" behind the heart. This backup of blood is called heart failure or congestion by physicians, and it produces a number of symptoms, such as shortness of breath, fatigue, poor appetite, and ankle swelling. Congestion, or heart failure, can be effectively combated with a number of medicines. The occurrence of heart failure is *not* a sign that the heart will soon cease to function. Effective therapy is available to reverse the circulatory changes of heart failure or congestion.

Heart attacks can also cause the heart muscle to become abnormally stiff, which can also cause blood to back up behind the heart, resulting in symptoms that resemble those of heart failure. This stiffening process is usually short-lived, disappearing three or four days after the onset of the heart attack.

The electrical system of the heart is very frequently disturbed following a myocardial infarction. The heart may exhibit a number of abnormal beating patterns and cardiac arrest can result. One of the functions of the coronary care unit is to watch closely for electrical disturbances so that appropriate treatment may be given to correct them. Most electrical disturbances of the heartbeat gradually disappear during the first week following a heart attack. Some disturbances may remain and these can often be combated with medication.

Scar formation in the area where a heart attack has occurred takes approximately three to six weeks. The resulting scar in the heart is a stiffened area of scar tissue minus heart muscle. The healing process is speeded or slowed according to a number of factors that include the severity of the attack, the age of the person having it, and the general health of the individual who suffered the attack. Since the rate of healing varies from person to person, return to activity will also vary from person to person, depending upon the speed of recovery. In most people who suffer a heart attack, the heart recovers sufficiently so that essentially all activities that were performed before the attack can be resumed after an appropriate healing period has passed. This is so because most people have considerably more heart muscle than is needed in order to perform their usual daily activities.

The critical phase of a heart attack occurs within the first few hours and days following the beginning of the episode. It is during this time that electrical complications, heart failure, and increased heart stiffness are common occurrences. It is clear, therefore, that these first few hours and days are best spent in the protective environment of a coronary care unit, where careful observation of the heart's activity can be made.

4.
Angina (Chest Discomfort) and Its Relation to Heart Attacks (Myocardial Infarctions)

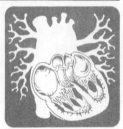

The deficiency of blood in the heart muscle that results from narrowing of the coronary arteries is particularly marked when the heart is called upon to increase its pumping activity. Increase in heart pumping activity occurs with exercise, a surge of emotion, psychological stress, or following eating. At such times, the patient with coronary atherosclerosis is most prone to note symptoms related to the deficiency of blood flow in his/her heart muscle. Two reactions may occur that reflect this deficiency of blood in the working heart muscle: angina pectoris or myocardial infarction.

Angina pectoris is a temporary chest discomfort that will cease when the additional work of the heart ceases or if an increased amount of blood can somehow be brought into the area of heart muscle that has the deficiency of blood flow. Thus, if an individual experiences angina pectoris while climbing the stairs, this amount of exercise is causing the heart to work harder and require more blood flow. Stressing a heart with narrowed arteries in this way results in a deficiency of blood in the heart muscle producing the symptom of angina pectoris. If the individual sits down to rest for a few moments, allowing the heart work to decrease, then the symptom of angina pectoris will also decrease. In summary, then, angina pectoris is due to a temporary lack of blood in the heart muscle that is brought on by increased work demands placed on the heart. Removal of this additional work load from the heart results in a complete annulment of the blood deficiency in the heart and a return to normal. The medication nitroglycerin may speed the recovery of the heart by relaxing the heart muscle, thereby decreasing the work of the heart and allowing dilation of the auxiliary blood vessels, which would in turn increase the blood flow into those areas of the heart that were suffering from a deficient blood supply.

Occasionally, an individual will experience angina pectoris without very much exertion or stress. In fact, angina may occur in the middle of the night and awaken the person from sleep. At other times, people notice that their angina, which had been fairly mild, has now become much more severe. Stresses that formerly did not bring it on may at a later date cause it to occur. This pattern of increasing angina pectoris, occurring with less and less exertion, results eventually in angina at rest or during sleep. It is called unstable angina because it is not responsive to activity levels and therefore can very easily proceed to myocardial infarction.

As mentioned earlier, angina pectoris and its underlying cause, inadequate blood flow to the heart muscle, are completely reversible. Myocardial infarction, however, represents actual death of heart cells and, as such, is not reversible.

The symptoms of angina pectoris and myocardial infarction may resemble each other. It is important to note, however, that each individual has his/her own pattern of discomfort. Some individuals may have predominant chest discomfort, while others may report predominant neck or arm discomfort. The list below includes possible manifestations of the anginal or myocardial infarction pain syndrome.

1. Many individuals report either a heaviness, burning, squeezing tightening, or pressure-like sensation in the middle of the chest, usually behind the breastbone. This sensation is rarely described as pain; it is more often described as discomfort.

2. This discomfort may spread to both arms, particularly the wrists, and up into the neck or jaw. It may also pass into the back. Occasionally, a person feels the discomfort only in the neck, jaw, back, or arms. Discomfort may occur in any combination of chest, arm, neck, jaw, or back location.

3. Numbness or tingling sensations may also occur in the shoulders, arms, wrists or fingers of individuals at the same time that the other discomforts described above occur.

4. If the pain is the result of angina pectoris, the discomfort usually increases if the stressful situation, such as exercise, continues, and decreases if the stressful factor is removed.

5. If it is due to angina, the discomfort usually fades away several minutes after the patient places a nitroglycerin tablet under the tongue.

6. The discomfort of myocardial infarction is very similar to that described above for angina pectoris, but it is more severe, lasts longer, and may be associ-

ated with sweating and nausea. The discomfort of angina pectoris rarely lasts longer than fifteen minutes, while that of myocardial infarction may last for several hours. The pain of myocardial infarction does not disappear with rest or nitroglycerin therapy.

7. The pain of angina pectoris or myocardial infarction does not increase when one takes a deep breath. (But see pericarditis, page 35.)

What should one do to relieve the discomfort of angina pectoris? First, cease all activity, sit down, and rest. If nitroglycerin has been prescribed, place one tablet under the tongue and allow it to dissolve. In almost all cases of angina pectoris, these two procedures will result in the disappearance of the discomfort within a few minutes. If the discomfort persists for more than five minutes, a second nitroglycerin tablet should be taken. If a second dose does not relieve or significantly diminish the discomfort, the individual should be taken to the nearest hospital emergency room.

Nitroglycerin is not habit forming. Moreover, the body does not become used to nitroglycerin and does not need progressively greater dosages to achieve the same relief. This means that if pain persists after two nitroglycerin tablets, the patient may take a third or even fourth tablet while preparations are under way for the drive to the hospital emergency room. The additional nitroglycerin tablets should be spaced at five- to ten-minute intervals, and the patient should not be lying down when taking the tablets (see Appendix D). If the pain increases following nitroglycerin or if the individual becomes light-headed, no further tablets should be taken.

It is important that nitroglycerin tablets be fresh, since they tend to lose their potency with age. Thus, the prescription should be refilled at least every six months. The drug should be kept in a tightly sealed brown glass bottle with the cotton removed.

Unlike a heart attack, angina is not life threatening. Many patients lead full, active lives despite daily bouts of angina pectoris. Only rarely (unless it is unstable) does angina proceed to myocardial infarction. In most instances, angina is rapidly relieved by rest and nitroglycerin.

What You Should Do if You Think You Are Having a Myocardial Infarction

As mentioned above, the discomfort of angina pectoris may closely resemble the discomfort of myocardial infarction. In fact, physicians distinguish between angina pectoris and myocardial infarction mainly by means of the duration of the discomfort. Thus, if the discomfort is short-lived, lasting only a few minutes, it is likely to be angina pectoris. If the discomfort is prolonged, it may very well be due to a myocardial infarction. When it is difficult to decide whether an individual has had a serious bout of angina pectoris or a myocardial infarction, the safest step is to admit the patient to the hospital and follow his/her electrocardiogram and blood tests to see whether, in fact, there has been any damage to the heart.

The discomfort of myocardial infarction is frequently more severe than that of angina pectoris, and many patients can distinguish clearly between their more mild, usual anginal pains and the more severe pain of myo-cardial infarction, even though both pains occur in simi-lar locations and have similar qualities. In particular, the discomfort associated with myocardial infarction can be accompanied by cold sweats, nausea, light-headedness, and a feeling of terror. Should one have these symptoms in association with chest discomfort, immediate plans should be made to get to the hospital emergency room.

Once the decision has been made to go to the emer-gency room, no unnecessary time should be lost getting there. Do not spend time trying to reach a physician. The patient should not drive. If no driver is near at hand, the person should call the police, an ambulance service, or a taxicab. It is preferable to call for medically trained personnel such as the police or fire department ambulance squad, rather than for a taxi. However, if a taxi is convenient and available, it would be better to take it immediately to the hospital emergency room rather than delaying to make a phone call and waiting for the police. Any delay may make the patient's condi-tion worse. If heart damage has occurred, time is precious. At the emergency room, electrocardiograms and a careful examination of the heart will be performed. Both of these help to determine whether the episode was just a bad bout of angina pectoris or whether indeed heart damage has occurred. If there is any doubt, the patient will be admitted to the hospital. Sometimes prolonged bouts of angina signal a need for change in the patient's medicines. In some cases bouts of angina indicate that the patient may require a heart operation known as coro-nary artery bypass grafting, discussed in Chapter 7.

Many patients delay inordinately following the onset

of symptoms that signal a myocardial infarction. There are many reasons for this. Some individuals do not want to disturb their family or friends. Others tell themselves that this pain is not really very much different from other discomforts they have had. Clearly, the physician cannot be of help in this situation. The patient must decide the appropriate time to come to the hospital. Let a word to the wise suffice here: no harm is done if one makes an occasional trip to the hospital emergency room and discovers that this episode of discomfort was due only to angina pectoris. Much harm may be done if one stays at home with a myocardial infarction.

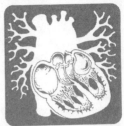

Coronary care units were first introduced to provide a special protective environment for patients who had suffered heart attacks. The term coronary care unit is frequently abbreviated as CCU in the slang of the hospital. The coronary care unit staff are specially trained to deal with heart attack patients, and they are aided by a great deal of sophisticated electronic equipment.

Patients are frequently afraid of the equipment when they first enter the coronary care unit. After staying in the unit for a period of time, however, most patients realize that the equipment is there to help them and that it is not threatening or in any way dangerous.

Small electrodes are placed on the chests of all patients when first admitted to the coronary care unit. These electrodes are often made of plastic or paper, and they help the physicians and nurses observe the electrical activity of the heart. They record a constant electrocardiogram, which is a record of the heart's electrical activity (Figure 5). Patients having heart attacks can have abnormalities in the electrical activity of their hearts

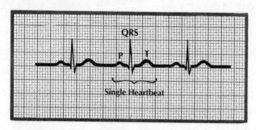

FIGURE 5. The Electrical Activity of the Heart

The electrical signal is recorded on an electrocardiogram or seen on a coronary care unit monitor screen. The part of the signal labeled P corresponds to electrical activity in the right and left atria. That part of the signal labeled QRS corresponds to right and left ventricular electrical activity. The part of the signal labeled T is electrical activity generated by the heart as it "resets" itself for the next beat.

(abnormal heart rhythm, or cardiac arrhythmia), and constant monitoring of this activity enables the doctors and nurses to identify and treat any electrical problems that arise. Patients may feel these abnormal heart rhythms as "skipped beats" or palpitations. Frequent blood pressure and pulse checks are made in the CCU.

A small needle or a small plastic tube called an I.V. is placed in the veins of all patients who are admitted to a coronary care unit. Through this needle or tube, sugar and water flow constantly, carrying various medications directly into the bloodstream. Some patients require considerable amounts of medicines administered intravenously, while others require almost none. A great number of different medications are given orally, intravenously, or as a paste spread on the skin to patients who have suffered myocardial infarctions. Some of these medicines are given around-the-clock, while others are given only intermittently or once a day. Many of these medications are discussed in Chapters 6 and 14 and Appendix C.

Frequent blood tests are performed in the coronary care unit. Damaged heart muscle releases a number of substances into the bloodstream. Some of these substances, called enzymes, can be measured by means of blood tests that help the physician detect and determine the extent of heart damage.

A number of highly sophisticated and specialized machines are used under special circumstances in the coronary care unit. These devices help to treat certain unusual problems that can arise. For example, the electrical cardioverter is used to deliver a significant electric shock to the heart. This electric shock treatment (cardioversion or defibrillation) may be necessary for patients who develop abnormal heartbeat rhythms (ventricular tachycardia, ventricular fibrillation). The individual who receives the shock is put to sleep with intravenous medication so that the discomfort associated with the shock is not felt.

Some patients require careful determination of the blood pressure within the heart itself. In order to do this, special tubes, or catheters, have been developed that can be inserted into the body and into the heart with a minimum of difficulty and a minimum of risk. These catheters are inserted through the skin after an anesthetic has been injected so that the procedure will not be uncomfortable for the patient. Catheters can be inserted into the body in a number of places including the neck, the arm, or the groin. The positioning of these catheters within the heart requires a skilled physician who follows the progress of the catheter's trip into the heart with an x-ray machine called a fluoroscope.

Some patients' hearts have abnormal electrical activity requiring regulation by a pacemaker. Pacemakers have wires that are inserted into the heart. The wires are passed into the heart through a vein in a manner similar to the insertion of an intravenous needle or a catheter. The x-ray fluoroscope machine is often employed to help position the pacemaker wire in the heart. The wire itself is then hooked to a small electrical device known as the pacemaker box, which is often attached to the patient's arm or leg with adhesive tape. This box generates electrical activity that helps to keep the heart beating regularly and at an appropriate rate. The electrical energy delivered to the heart by a pacemaker is many thousands of times less than that delivered by the electrical cardioverter mentioned earlier.

Occasionally, patients require the therapeutic assistance of the balloon pump. This is a slender, sausage-shaped device, approximately a foot long, that increases blood flow in the heart while helping the heart muscle to work. It is inserted into the aorta, the main blood vessel leaving the heart. The balloon is inflated and deflated electronically with helium or carbon dioxide gas during each cardiac cycle. Inflation of the balloon increases blood flow through narrowed coronary arteries; deflation helps the left ventricular pumping chamber to deliver blood to the body. Placing this pump in the body is a job performed by a vascular surgeon. It requires an operation on the groin, where the balloon is inserted into an artery. This operation and other small operations can be performed in the coronary care unit after anesthetic, or nerve-deadening medicine, has been injected into the skin. Although the injection of the anesthetic causes temporary discomfort, the medication protects the patient against severe pain during these minor operations.

Rarely, patients experience severe breathing difficulties during recovery from a heart attack. In such instances it may be necessary to place a tube in the patient's windpipe. This tube is connected to a respirator, which pumps air into the lungs at regular intervals, helping the patient to breathe. An adequate supply of oxygen is ensured until recovery enables the patient to breathe unaided.

6.
Hospital Treatment: Pain, Abnormal Heart Rhythm, Heart Failure

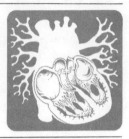

A number of different problems can occur in heart attack patients, requiring a number of different treatments. Following are some of the problems and the treatments for them.

Treatment of Pain

Patients who suffer myocardial infarction frequently come to the hospital because of pain. Some individuals will find that this chest, arm, neck, or back discomfort has disappeared by the time they arrive at the hospital emergency room. Others, however, will continue to feel considerable discomfort even after being admitted to the coronary care unit. There are a number of different medicines that help to control the patient's discomfort. The most well known, and frequently the most effective medication for control of pain, is morphine. Morphine and its first cousin, meperidine (Demerol), are opiate narcotics. Both are extremely effective painkillers and are usually given to the patient intravenously. In some coronary care units, patients breathe a mixture of oxygen and laughing gas (nitrous oxide), which also helps relieve any pain they might feel. A mild sedative such as diazepam (Valium) is usually also prescribed for patients who have myocardial infarction. Such sedation helps relieve both physical and psychological discomfort.

Sometimes the pericardium, the membrane surrounding the heart, becomes inflamed. This irritation, known as pericarditis, can be quite painful, particularly when the patient takes a deep breath. The discomfort associated with pericarditis is often effectively treated with repeated doses of aspirin or indomethacin (Indocin).

Treatment of Electrical Problems

Patients who suffer a myocardial infarction frequently have problems associated with the electrical system in their hearts. A number of different kinds of electrical disturbance (arrhythmia, dysrhythmia) can occur. One type consists of "runaway" heart rhythm (tachycardia) in which the heart beats much too fast to be efficient. The heartbeat may be regular or irregular. As a result of tachycardia, patients may experience palpitations, chest discomfort, or shortness of breath. Another form of electrical disturbance is a kind of short circuit in the transmission of electrical impulses in the heart, causing the heartbeat to be too slow for the heart to function efficiently. Such a slow heart rate (bradycardia) may also be regular or irregular.

Three forms of therapy are used in the coronary care unit to treat these electrical difficulties. The first form of therapy involves the administration of anti-arrhythmic medication, intravenously or orally, to stop or consider-ably improve electrical difficulties. Some of these medications are lidocaine (Xylocaine), procainamide (Pronestyl), quinidine, propranolol (Inderal), and di-phenylhydantoin (Dilantin). They are used alone or in combination to stop abnormal heartbeat rhythms. If medications are ineffective in abolishing cardiac arrhyth-mias, or if the arrhythmia is life-threatening, electric shock (defibrillation or cardioversion) may be used to terminate the abnormal heart rhythm. During defibrilla-tion, a large electric shock is delivered at any point in the course of the cardiac cycle. During cardioversion, however, smaller shocks are delivered in a particular phase of the cardiac cycle. Defibrillation is usually used to reverse a cardiac arrest and it is hence an emergency procedure. Cardioversion is used to reverse more benign abnormalities of the heartbeat, is not an emergency pro-cedure, and is usually performed at the patient's con-venience.

When the heartbeat rhythm is too slow for the heart to function efficiently, an electric pacemaker, described in Chapter 8, can be wired into the heart. Some patients require a permanent electric pacemaker, placed under the skin of the chest. Most individuals who require a pacemaker in the coronary care unit, however, only need this form of therapy temporarily. After a period of sev-eral days, the pacemaker can be removed because the heart has corrected the abnormal electrical short circuit.

Sometimes, patients who have coronary artery disease, but no heart attack, die suddenly because of abnormal heartbeats (ventricular fibrillation). Certain tests (ex-ercise test, Holter monitor), anti-arrhythmic drugs, and pacemakers are used to evaluate and prevent this feared complication. Unfortunately, as with sexual matters, many patients are fearful of discussing sudden death with their doctor. Clearly, it is best to discuss these anxieties openly with the physician.

Treatment of Heart Failure (Congestion)

It is not uncommon for patients to develop some temporary heart failure (congestion) during the first few days or weeks after a heart attack. Congestion occurs because the heart muscle pumps less efficiently than it should. As mentioned earlier, the decreased strength of the heart muscle results in a "backup" of blood behind the heart. This back pressure causes the blood vessels in the lungs to become overdistended with blood, and such overdistended vessels can leak fluid into the lung tissue itself. In turn, fluid in the lungs interferes with normal breathing and makes the patient short of breath.

A number of medications are used to combat congestion (heart failure). These include digitalis preparations, which strengthen the heartbeat, and diuretic preparations, which remove excess fluid from the lungs and body by increasing the production of urine by the kidneys. The latest treatment for heart failure includes a number of medications (such as hydralazine or nitrates) that decrease blood pressure slightly and thereby reduce the work of the heart.

Sometimes it may be difficult to decide whether or not heart failure is present. In such a situation, it is frequently helpful to measure the blood pressure within the heart chambers themselves by placing a small tube, or catheter, in the heart, as described in the last chapter. Occasionally, a patient with heart failure benefits from the insertion of the balloon pump, also described in the last chapter. This device is used when medications have not adequately cleared the lungs of the excess fluid that may occur with heart failure. The balloon pump assists the heart's pumping action and thereby reduces the "backup" of blood into the lungs.

Treatment of Complications of Myocardial Infarction

For some patients, blood clots seem to play a role in either the heart attack or in complications following the myocardial infarction, and it may be necessary to administer blood thinners, or anticoagulants. There are two kinds of blood thinner. The first type, heparin, can be given only by injection, either beneath the skin or within a vein (intravenously). The second, oral blood thinners, may be prescribed for a number of months following a myocardial infarction. The oral blood thinner most commonly prescribed is warfarin (Coumadin). Patients taking this drug require periodic blood tests so that doses of the drug may be adjusted to ensure that exactly the correct amount is being taken.

Oxygen is almost always given to patients who have suffered a myocardial infarction. Oxygen therapy helps to decrease the work of the heart, and it may even decrease the extent of a heart attack. Oxygen is delivered either through small nasal tubes or by face mask.

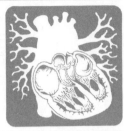

During the last ten years, some patients suffering from coronary artery disease have been treated with a highly effective operation known as coronary artery bypass. During this operation, an expendable vein is removed from the leg and sewn into the heart. This vein functions the same way as a detour on a highway that carries traffic around an obstruction in the road. The vein carries blood to the heart muscle, bypassing areas of narrowing in the coronary arteries (Figure 6). The operation is done with the heart stopped, and the body is supplied with nourishing blood by a pumping device known as the heart-lung machine.

Coronary artery bypass has become the commonest major operation in the United States today. It is usually very safe; during the procedure the risk of dying is 1 to 5 percent, and the risk of having a heart attack is 10 to 15 percent. Approximately 80 percent of the grafts remain functional one to five years after the operation. The grafts are able to supply the heart with approximately the same amount of blood as a normal artery. Coronary

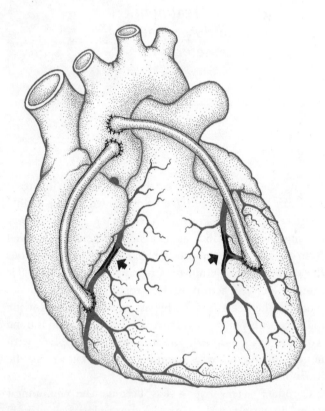

FIGURE 6. Bypass Grafts

Two coronary artery bypass grafts, to the anterior descending and the right coronary arteries. Note that the grafts are sewn at one end into the coronary arteries beyond areas of narrowing and at the other end into the aorta.

artery bypass is extremely effective in relieving patients of the discomfort of angina pectoris. Approximately 90 percent of individuals who have had this operation suffer little or no angina afterwards. The operation does not cure atherosclerosis, however. The underlying atherosclerotic process may continue to narrow other coronary arteries, and some patients experience the return of angina pectoris and even myocardial infarction.

Some patients with very severe coronary artery disease may live longer after having a coronary artery bypass, but most patients only obtain relief from angina pectoris. Many studies have shown that patients who undergo coronary artery bypass do not decrease their risk of having a fatal or nonfatal heart attack. However, surgically treated patients are usually able to lead more active lives than comparable medically treated patients because, as already noted, surgery almost always relieves angina pectoris.

Shortness of breath is usually a symptom of heart failure (failure of the heart to pump enough blood) in patients who have had a heart attack. Coronary artery bypass is usually ineffective in improving heart failure, and therefore the operation rarely relieves shortness of breath. In addition, this type of surgery carries larger risk for patients who have heart failure than for those who do not.

There is considerable disagreement among cardiologists about when to use surgical or medical therapy. In general, surgical therapy is advised when angina pectoris interferes with normal daily activities or when it occurs with little or no exertion. Often medical therapy is tried first. If medicines fail to control symptoms adequately, surgery may be advised. Coronary artery bypass surgery is rarely performed on individuals who have recently had a heart attack. Usually, two to three months are allowed to elapse between a myocardial infarction and cardiac surgery.

Occasionally, a heart attack results in severe damage to one of the walls of the heart or to one of the heart valves. Although such complications are unusual, they can cause considerable difficulty for the patient and are often best treated surgically.

Before heart surgery can be performed, it is almost always necessary to prepare a "road map" (angiogram) for the surgeon. Such preparations are made by a cardiologist during a procedure known as cardiac catheterization. During this minor operation, small plastic tubes (catheters) are passed through the skin (made numb by injected anesthetic) into blood vessels and from there into the heart. Dye, which appears on x-ray film, is injected into the heart chambers and arteries through the catheters. X-ray photos or movies (the angiograms mentioned above) are made while the dye is being injected. When such films are developed, they show the cardiologist and the cardiac surgeon the location of cardiac abnormalities that may be corrected by surgery.

8.
Pacemakers

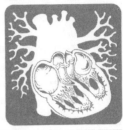

On occasion, a heart attack damages the "wiring" of the electrical system within the heart. In such cases, the heartbeat may slow markedly, and it may be necessary to insert a wire (a pacing catheter) into the heart and to supply the heart muscle with regular electrical stimulation from a specially designed battery-operated instrument (pacemaker generator). Some pacemakers may only be needed temporarily; others may be permanently implanted under the skin of the chest or abdomen (Figure 7).

Permanent pacemakers (wire and generator) are usually inserted during a brief operation. A number of different systems are available, all of which are quite reliable. Periodically, the batteries in the pacemaker generator become exhausted and must be replaced. Replacement occurs every three to four years and requires a small operation and brief hospitalization to replace the pacemaker generator, which is just beneath the skin.

Special devices exist to check on the function of a pacemaker after it has been inserted into the body. Pacemaker patients return every few months to have a "check up" of their pacemakers. Like any electrical device, pacemakers are prone to technical problems. Sometimes these can be solved without removing the pacemaker, but often it is necessary to replace the malfunctioning pacemaker with a new one.

In the past, patients who had pacemakers had to avoid close contact with certain electrical devices. Present-day pacemakers are electrically shielded in such a way that avoidance of electrical machinery is no longer necessary.

Most pacemakers do not function continuously. They operate only occasionally, when the heartbeat slows. In most cases, pacemakers improve the patient's sense of well-being. Malfunction of the pacemaker rarely threatens the patient's life, since most individuals have enough function left in the electrical system of the heart to get help in time.

FIGURE 7. Pacemaker

There are two methods of connecting a pacemaker to the heart. The first and most common is to insert the leads through a vein and have them go to the inside of the right ventricle, as in A. The other method involves attaching them to the outside of the right ventricle, as in B. The pulse generator, which contains the batteries, is located just under the skin of the abdomen or near the collarbone, as indicated.

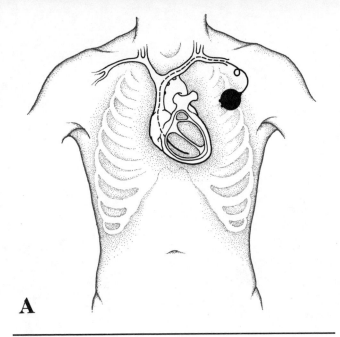

A

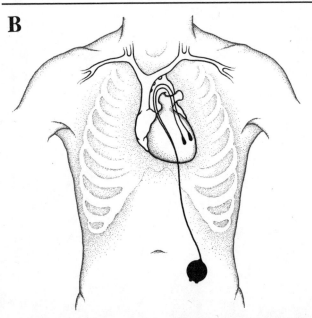

B

Part 2.
RECOVERY
AND STAYING WELL

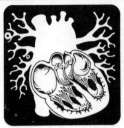

9.
Diet and Heart Disease

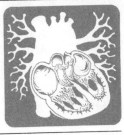

Two factors in the American diet contribute to the large number of heart attacks in the United States. Together, saturated fats and cholesterol are one of these factors. Saturated fat and cholesterol are two forms of fat that come from animal sources. They are present in large quantities in egg yolks, well-marbled meats, bacon, cream, and milk products having high butterfat content, such as butter and cheese. An individual's intake of saturated fat and cholesterol is directly related to his/her blood cholesterol level. Most researchers agree that the average American diet, heavy in calories and fat, contributes to the development of coronary atherosclerosis. The more cholesterol and saturated fat one eats, the larger will be the amount of cholesterol in the blood.

Overeating is the other dietary factor that hastens the development of coronary atherosclerosis. The average American diet leads not only to obesity but also to high blood fat levels (cholesterol and triglycerides), both of which speed the development of atherosclerosis and increase the risk of infarction. Moreover, extra pounds represent an extra work load for the heart that may already be getting insufficient quantities of nourishing blood. It is clear that an increase in the heart's work load in the face of a decreasing fuel supply can result in a dangerous imbalance of supply and demand within the heart muscle itself. One of the simplest methods for decreasing the work load of the heart is to reduce excess weight by dieting.

It is prudent for the patient who has suffered a heart attack to reduce his/her weight to the recommended value for his/her age and sex (see Table 2, pages 64–65). In addition, it would be wise to decrease significantly the intake of foods known to be rich in saturated fat. The diet described below is based on recent recommendations of the American Heart Association. It emphasizes decreased cholesterol and saturated fat ingestion in combination with increased intake of polyunsaturated fats.

Some patients with hereditary predisposition for markedly elevated blood cholesterol and/or triglyceride levels may require a more stringent diet, medications, and, rarely, an intestinal operation in order to lower the level of these fatty substances in the blood.

DEFINITIONS

Polyunsaturated Fat   is usually a fat of plant origin. Most liquid vegetable fats are unsaturated. Some are more unsaturated than others. For example: safflower and corn oil are more unsaturated than olive oil and peanut oil.

Saturated Fat	is usually a fat of animal origin; however, a solid vegetable shortening (hydrogenated) may be high in saturated fat. Coconut oil is also a saturated fat.
Cholesterol	is a fatty substance found in the blood, manufactured by the body. It is present in foods of animal origin.
Triglyceride	is a fatty substance found in the blood, absorbed directly from digested food and produced by the body from carbohydrates in the diet.

With this new diet it is necessary to make some changes in eating habits. Here are some suggestions for a wholesome diet that is low in cholesterol and saturated fat:

Eliminate foods that are high in cholesterol. These foods include egg yolk; shellfish; dairy products containing fat; baked goods prepared with egg yolk, butter, and whole milk; and organ meats such as heart, brain, kidney, liver, and sweetbreads.

Eliminate foods high in saturated fat, for example, animal fats such as lard, suet, salt pork, and bacon drippings. Solid vegetable shortenings should be avoided because hydrogenation increases the saturation of fats.

MEAT AND FAT IN THE DIET

To restrict the intake of saturated fat, many doctors recommend limiting the amount of meat in the diet.

The following amounts will provide the recommended portions:

1. Limit all meat, including fish and poultry, to no more than nine ounces of cooked meat per day, for example, two large hamburgers.
2. Limit beef, lamb, ham, and pork to three-ounce portions three times per week. Fish and poultry (without skin) are naturally lower in fat and should be used in place of meat as often as possible.
3. Try to use polyunsaturated fat whenever possible. The polyunsaturated fat (margarine and oil) does not have to be used during the same meal with meat. Use as much polyunsaturated fat as desired. It is not required, however, for one to eat excessive amounts of unsaturated fat. When oil or margarine is called for, try to employ products that contain unsaturated fat. The following suggestions are offered.

WAYS OF USING POLYUNSATURATED OIL

In food preparation:
> Broiling, baking, or frying meats, fish, and poultry
> Popping corn

As an ingredient:
> Salad dressings
> Barbecue sauces
> Cream sauces made with skim milk
> Marinades
> Pie crust
> Cakes and cookies made with skim milk and egg whites
> Cooked vegetable seasoning (add spices, herbs, etc.)

ESTIMATING MEAT, FISH, AND POULTRY PORTIONS

There are sixteen ounces to a pound. Raw meat, fish, or poultry lose weight when they are cooked.

Three ounces of cooked meat equals the following:
1) Four (4) ounces of raw meat or fish without bone
2) Three-fourths (¾) cup cooked, flaked, or chopped meat, poultry, or fish
3) A ground beef patty, 3″ diameter x 1″ thickness, cooked
4) One-half large chicken breast, cooked
5) One chicken thigh plus one drumstick, cooked

BUYING AND COOKING MEAT, FISH, AND POULTRY

Fish and poultry should be used in place of meat as often as possible. Try to eat meat, fish, and poultry only once a day. Eat meat only three days a week, using fish, poultry, or vegetarian main courses the rest of the week. Select cuts that look lean, that is, those having more muscle than fat. Avoid cuts of meat where the fat is distributed throughout (marbled) and cannot be removed. "Prime" grade meat is the most heavily marbled. Lower grades of meat are less heavily marbled and therefore contain less fat. Some stores now market packaged ground beef with the fat content clearly indicated. Use lean or very lean hamburger, or any other lean cut trimmed and ground to order, rather than regular ground hamburger, which is usually high in fat. Trim the fat from the meat selected and remove the skin from poultry.

Conventional cooking methods such as barbecuing and pan and oven broiling are particularly effective in reducing the fat from meat, fish, or poultry. Fat will drain from roasted or baked meat placed on a rack. The fat can be removed from the meat drippings by refrigerating the drippings until the fat has hardened. The fat can then be removed and discarded, and the rest of the drippings used for gravies. Or, instead of gravy, safflower oil or margarine can be used.

LEARNING TO LIVE WITH THE DIET

Cutting down on fats in the diet requires only a small adjustment in taste for the dieter. Oriental cuisine is an example that low-fat cooking can be rich in variety and flavor. Many cookbooks, newspapers, and magazines now publish recipes using the proper foods and fats to create good meals.*

The contents of packaged foods are marked on the label. It is important to note that a label listing "vegetable fat" or "containing no animal fat" or "nondairy" does not necessarily mean that the product contains polyunsaturated fat. Such a label might refer to coconut oil or hydrogenated vegetable fat — both of which are to be avoided. If weight is a problem and calories are being counted, be sure to consult the dietitian or physician for assistance.

* See R. Eshleman and M. Winston, eds., *American Heart Association Cookbook* (New York: David McKay, 1973).

LOW CHOLESTEROL,
LOW SATURATED FAT DIET

Type of Food	Included	Excluded
Beverages (nondairy)	Coffee, tea, carbonated beverages, fruit and vegetable juice.	None
Breads	Whole wheat, rye, or white bread, matzo, saltines, and graham crackers. Baked goods containing no whole milk or egg yolk and made with allowed fat.	Biscuits, commercial muffins, sweet rolls, cornbread, pancakes, waffles, french toast, hot rolls, corn chips, potato chips, cheese crackers or other flavored crackers.
Cereals	All cereals; also grain products such as rice, macaroni, noodles, spaghetti, and flour.	None
Dairy Products	Skim milk, nonfat buttermilk, dried nonfat milk, evaporated skim milk, dry (no-fat) cottage cheese, yogurt made from skim milk, skim milk cheese such as Sapsago.	Whole milk, whole milk drinks, dried whole milk, evaporated milk, condensed milk, cream (sweet or sour), ice cream, ice milk, sherbet, commercial whipped toppings, cream substitutes, cream cheese, all hard cheese except skim milk cheese, creamed cottage

Type of Food	Included	Excluded
		cheese unless substituted for meat. One-fourth cup creamed cottage cheese equals 1 ounce of meat.
Desserts	Fruit ices (water ices) ; angel food cake including angel food cake mix; puddings made with skim milk; gelatins; frostings made with allowed fat; meringues; cakes, cookies, and pies made with allowed fats and skim milk (no egg yolks) ; fruit whips; junkets made with skim milk.	Desserts that contain whole milk, saturated or hydrogenated fat, and egg yolks, including commercial pies, cakes, and cookies; all cake and cookie mixes (except angel food cake mixes) .
Fats	Safflower oil, corn oil, soft safflower margarine* and commercial mayonnaise. *Liquid safflower oil —not hardened, partially hardened, or hydrogenated—should be the first listed ingredient. (The first listed item on the label indicates the predominant ingredient.)	Butter, lard, hydrogenated margarine and shortening, coconut oil, and all other oils not listed; salt pork, suet, bacon, and meat drippings; gravies unless made with allowed polyunsaturated fat; sauces, such as cream sauce, etc., unless made with allowed fat and skim milk.

Type of Food	Included	Excluded
Fruit	Any fresh, canned, frozen, or dried fruit or juice. Avocado may be used in small amounts.	None
Meat, Poultry, Fish	*Limit as recommended:* Lean beef, lamb, veal, pork and ham, tongue, chicken, turkey, dried or chipped beef, fish except those excluded, egg white, and peanut butter.	Egg yolk; luncheon meat; cold cuts; hot dogs; sausages; bacon; goose; duck; poultry skin; shellfish including oysters, lobster, scallops, shrimp, clams, and crab; fish roe including caviar; all organ meats such as heart, liver, brains, and kidney; all fatty meats; regular fried meats and fried fish unless fried with allowed oils; corned beef; *regular* ground beef or hamburger; spareribs; pork and beans; meats canned or frozen in sauces or gravies; frozen or packaged dinners; frozen or packaged prepared products (convenience foods).
Soups	Bouillon, clear broth, fat free vegetable soup, cream	All others.

Type of Food	Included	Excluded
	soup made with skim milk, packaged dehydrated soups.	
Sweets	Hard candies, jam, jelly, honey, sugar, syrup containing no fat.	All other candies or chocolates.
Vegetables	Any fresh, frozen, or canned, cooked without saturated fat.	Buttered, creamed, or fried vegetables unless prepared with allowed fat.
Miscellaneous	Olives, pickles, salt, spices, herbs, nuts, except those excluded, and cocoa.	Coconut, cashew, and macadamia nuts.

The menu patterns on page 61 are recommended guides for planning meals that will provide the necessary nutrients.

The following guide includes suggestions on how to select foods when eating away from home.

SUGGESTIONS FOR MEALS AWAY FROM HOME

Many dieters purchase one or more meals a week in a restaurant. A dieter may find that his/her special needs get more attention at a certain restaurant. A regular customer can ask for foods prepared in the special low fat cooking method.

Meat: Ask that all meat fat be trimmed. The meal can consist of a chop, steak, chicken, or fish. Request the

SAMPLE MENU PATTERN *(1700–2000 Calories)*

Daily Food Plan	*Sample Menu Pattern*
1 pint or more skim milk	**BREAKFAST**
Cooked poultry, fish or lean trimmed meat	Citrus fruit or juice Cereal Toast
5 servings of vegetable and fruit; include:	Allowed fat Jelly and sugar
1 serving citrus fruit*	Skim milk
1 serving dark-green or	Coffee or tea if desired
deep-yellow vegetable†	**LUNCH**
7 or more servings of whole grained or enriched bread or cereal‡	Poultry, fish, or lean meat Potato or substitute
1 or more servings of potato, rice, etc.	Vegetables Bread
Allowed fat	Allowed fat Fruit or allowed dessert Skim milk
Allowed desserts and sweets	**DINNER**
	Poultry, fish, or lean meat Potato or substitute
	Vegetable
	Bread Allowed fat Fruit or allowed dessert Skim milk
	BETWEEN MEAL SNACK Fruit Skim milk

* One serving of citrus fruit daily is recommended to provide adequate vitamin C.
† One dark-green or deep-yellow vegetable is recommended daily to provide adequate vitamin A.
‡ Enriched cereal or bread should be included in the diet to provide adequate vitamin B complex and iron.

meat be broiled *without fat*. Limit the amount and kind of meat according to your diet plan.

Vegetable: Any vegetable prepared without fat may be included. No vegetables that are creamed or prepared in a sauce containing fat, whole milk, or cheese may be used.

Salad: Most ingredients such as vegetables, fruit or gelatin are allowed on your diet. Avoid cheese, including cream cheese, sour cream, or whipped cream. Select a salad dressing such as Italian, French, or oil and vinegar if the waiter indicates that an oil allowed on your diet (safflower, peanut, corn) has been used in the dressing. Often lemon or vinegar dressing is the wisest choice.

Fat: Margarine, salad dressings, and so on, listed in the diet may be selected.

Bread: Saltines are usually available. In addition, plain sliced bread and hard rolls may be eaten. Avoid hot rolls, biscuits, cornbread, popovers, muffins, etc., because all of these will contain fat that might be saturated. Sugar, jams, jellies, etc., may be eaten as desired.

Beverage: Skim milk is frequently available. Coffee or tea, fruit or vegetable juice, or a sweetened beverage (cola, etc.) are all allowed.

Dessert: Fruit and Jell-O are listed on most menus; angel food cake and fruit ice may be available. Avoid any dessert that might contain ingredients not allowed on the diet, such as fat, egg yolk, whole milk, or whipped cream.

SALT IN THE DIET

Some patients may be restricted by their physicians in the amount of salt allowed in their diet. This is usually the case if the individual is suffering from high blood pressure or heart failure. The following foods* are high in salt content and should be avoided by persons on a salt (or sodium) restricted diet.

Any commercial foods made of whole milk: ice cream, sherbet, milk shakes, chocolate milk, malted milk, milk mixes, condensed milk, instant cocoa mixes, and other beverage mixes

Commercial candies

Baking soda (sodium bicarbonate)

Pudding mixes

Yeast breads or rolls or melba toast made with salt or from commercial mixes

Quick breads made with baking powder, baking soda, or salt, or made from commercial mixes

Salted popcorn, potato chips, pretzels, and other "snack" foods

Canned, salted, or smoked meat: bacon, bologna, chipped or corned beef, frankfurters, ham, kosher meats, luncheon meats, salt pork, sausage, smoked tongue, etc.

Frozen fish fillets

* Modified from D. S. Frederickson, R. I. Levy, E. Jones, et al. *Dietary Management of Hyperlipoproteinemia: A Handbook for Physicians*, NHL 1, Bethesda, Maryland, 1970.

Canned, salted, or smoked fish: anchovies, caviar, salted and dried cod, herring, canned salmon, sardines, canned tuna, etc.

Peanut butter

Salted butter

Bacon and bacon fat

Olives, pickles, and relishes

Salt pork

Commercial French or other dressings

Salted margarine

Salted nuts

Canned vegetables or vegetable juices except low-sodium dietetic

Sauerkraut

Catsup, chili sauce, mustard (prepared), horse-radish (prepared)

Celery leaves, dried or fresh, celery salt, celery seed, garlic salt, onion salt

Meat extracts, meat sauces, tenderizers, bouillon cubes, monosodium glutamate, Worcestershire sauce, soy sauce

Salt

Use of Alcohol after a Myocardial Infarction

Alcohol is a mild poison for the heart muscle. Consequently, patients who have heart disease of any kind should use alcoholic beverages only moderately. Doctors recognize that many individuals enjoy relaxing with a pre-dinner cocktail or a glass or two of wine with their meals. Prohibiting such a moderate intake of alcohol might occasion tension or distress more harmful to the heart than the modest quantity of alcohol imbibed.

Most physicians urge sparing use of alcohol for all their patients, including heart attack patients. Total abstinence is usually not necessary after a myocardial infarction. It should be noted, however, that individuals whose heart attacks have resulted in the development of heart failure may be particularly susceptible to the adverse effects of alcohol on the heart. Such individuals should be particularly temperate in their use of alcoholic beverages. In general, one or two medium-strength cocktails, or two to three glasses of beer or wine per day will not significantly damage the heart of a patient who has suffered a myocardial infarction.

TABLE 2. *Desirable Weights of Adults**

Desirable weight (in indoor clothing), ages 25 and over

Height (in shoes)			SMALL FRAME		MEDIUM FRAME		LARGE FRAME	
ft in		cm	lb	kg	lb	kg	lb	kg
					MEN			
5 2		157.5	112–120	50.8–54.4	118–129	53.5–58.5	126–141	57.2–64
5 3		160	115–123	52.2–55.8	121–133	54.9–60.3	129–144	58.5–65.3
5 4		162.6	118–126	53.5–57.2	124–136	56.2–61.7	132–148	59.9–67.1
5 5		165.1	121–129	54.9–58.5	127–139	57.6–63	135–152	61.2–68.9
5 6		167.6	124–133	56.2–60.3	130–143	59 –64.9	138–156	62.6–70.8
5 7		170.2	128–137	58.1–62.1	134–147	60.8–66.7	142–161	64.4–73
5 8		172.7	132–141	59.9–64	138–152	62.6–68.9	147–166	66.7–75.3
5 9		175.3	136–145	61.7–65.8	142–156	64.4–70.8	151–170	68.5–77.1
5 10		177.8	140–150	63.5–68	146–160	66.2–72.6	155–174	70.3–78.9
5 11		180.3	144–154	65.3–69.9	150–165	68 –74.8	159–179	72.1–81.2
6 0		182.9	148–158	67.1–71.7	154–170	69.9–77.1	164–184	74.4–83.5
6 1		185.4	152–162	68.9–73.5	158–175	71.7–79.4	168–189	76.2–85.7
6 2		188	156–167	70.8–75.7	162–180	73.5–81.6	173–194	78.5–88
6 3		190.5	160–171	72.6–77.6	167–185	75.7–83.5	178–199	80.7–90.3
6 4		193	164–175	74.4–79.4	172–190	78.1–86.2	182–204	82.7–92.5

WOMEN

4	10	147.3	41.7–44.5	92– 98	43.5–48.5	96–107	47.2–54	104–119
4	11	149.9	42.6–45.8	94–101	44.5–49.9	98–110	48.1–55.3	106–122
5	0	152.4	43.5–47.2	96–104	45.8–51.3	101–113	49.4–56.7	109–125
5	1	154.9	44.9–48.5	99–107	47.2–52.6	104–116	50.8–58.1	112–128
5	2	157.5	46.3–49.9	102–110	48.5–54	107–119	52.2–59.4	115–131
5	3	160	47.6–51.3	105–113	49.9–55.3	110–122	53.5–60.8	118–134
5	4	162.6	49 –52.6	108–116	51.3–57.2	113–126	54.9–62.6	121–138
5	5	165.1	50.3–54	111–119	49 –59	116–130	49.4–64.4	125–142
5	6	167.6	51.7–55.8	114–123	54.4–61.2	120–135	58.5–66.2	129–146
5	7	170.2	53.5–57.6	118–127	56.2–63	124–139	60.3–68	133–150
5	8	172.7	55.3–59.4	122–131	58.1–64.9	128–143	62.1–69.9	137–154
5	9	175.3	57.2–61.2	126–135	59.9–66.7	132–147	64 –71.7	141–158
5	10	177.8	59 –63.5	130–140	61.7–68.5	136–151	65.8–73.9	145–163
5	11	180.3	60.8–65.3	134–144	63.5–70.3	140–155	67.6–76.2	149–168
6	0	182.9	62.6–67.1	138–148	65.3–72.1	144–159	69.4–78.5	153–173

* Weights of insured persons in the United States associated with lowest mortality. From *Metropolitan Life Insurance Company Statistical Bulletin*, 40, Nov.–Dec. 1959.

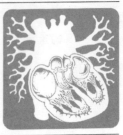

Cigarette smoking is the risk factor most often associated with heart attacks in the United States. Although not conclusively proven, the link between heart disease (and cancer) and cigarettes is so strong that the Surgeon General of the United States has instructed that a warning against the dangers of smoking be printed on every package of cigarettes. A number of scientists believe that substances that enter the blood during smoking actually cause damage to the linings of blood vessels in the heart. This allows cholesterol and other fatty substances to enter the blood vessel wall, thereby speeding the process that may eventually lead to myocardial infarction.

A cigarette smoker has a constant level of carbon monoxide, a poisonous gas, in his/her bloodstream. Carbon monoxide combines with hemoglobin in the blood, thus preventing the blood cells from carrying the normal quantity of life-giving oxygen. If an individual has narrowings in the coronary arteries, further impairment in the oxygen supply to the heart muscle resulting from carbon monoxide in the blood could be dangerous.

Thus, cigarette smoking both speeds the development of coronary atherosclerosis and decreases the nourishing abilities of the blood, two factors that can hasten the development of a heart attack.

Cigarette smoking would seem to be the major offender in increasing the risk of myocardial infarction. Cigar and pipe smoking have been shown to have little or no damaging effects on the heart. It would seem reasonable, however, that cigar and pipe smokers who inhale tobacco smoke also increase their risk of developing a myocardial infarction. Given the other dangers to your health that smoking involves in addition to its contribution to heart disease, it can only make sense not to smoke if at all possible.

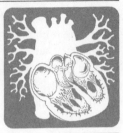

The severity of a heart attack, healing rate, and general strength and stamina vary from person to person. Consequently, the period of time it takes to recuperate after a myocardial infarction will vary also. A previously healthy individual who suffers a small heart attack might return to full activity within four to six weeks. On the other hand, a person having a larger heart attack, or one experiencing other health problems as well, may require a convalescence period of three to six months. Most patients feel tired and weak for a number of weeks and even for several months, due both to the weakness of their heart and inactivity during convalescence. Such persons need plenty of rest for the healing process to be effective.

There are three phases of recuperation for patients who have suffered a heart attack. Phase one takes place in the coronary care unit. The patient spends most of the day in bed with daily periods of sitting in a chair. He or she also gets out of bed to use a bedside commode or nearby toilet. This phase lasts from three to seven days. It is followed by phase two, during which time the patient is transferred to the regular hospital floor or to an intermediate coronary care area. Here, progressive increases in daily activity occur. At first, only small amounts of walking within the room are allowed. As the patient regains strength and the heart heals, more and more walking is done, both in the room and in the hallways. Phase two of the recuperative process lasts from two to ten days. During phase three, patients are prepared for discharge from the hospital. They are now in an ordinary hospital room. Increased activity is allowed. Phase three of recovery continues after the patient has been discharged from the hospital. The in-hospital part of this phase lasts from five to ten days while the outpatient part may last weeks or months. Activity is gradually increased throughout this period of time.

Some physicians have their patients count their pulse rates to measure how hard the heart works. The more strenuous a particular activity is, the faster the heart rate. Early in phase three, no activity should be performed that increases the heart rate to more than 100 to 110 beats per minute. Late in phase three, patients are allowed to achieve heart rates in the range of 120 to 130 beats per minute.

Some physicians have their patients perform bicycle or treadmill exercise tests at periodic intervals to evaluate the heart's response to exercise. The exercise test is used to judge when and if more strenuous activity can be undertaken.

The "Mets" (metabolic) system for measuring the strenuousness of work is used in many cardiac rehabilitation centers. A Met is a measure of work. One Met equals the amount of energy used while sitting quietly in a chair. All other activities are compared to chair-sitting and given different values on the Met scale depending on how strenuous they are. Thus, the more strenuous an activity, the higher will be its Met rating. Physicians using this system give their patients a list of the Met costs of different activities and tell them how many Mets the patient may perform during the various phases of the rehabilitation program. In other words, if a patient is allowed to perform activities of up to 3 Mets, this means that he is allowed to participate in activities whose strenuousness is 3 Mets or less. Typically, patients are allowed up to 3.5 Mets early in the recovery period for a heart attack (three to six weeks after myocardial infarction). Even more strenuous activity may be allowed at a later date, particularly if the patient is involved in a program of physical training. Approximate Met equivalents for a number of activities are listed in Table 3.

Returning to Work

After a two to three month recovery phase, most individuals will be able to return to previous levels of work and recreation. Many physicians use exercise tests and/or small continuously recording electrocardiogram machines known as Holter monitors to judge when an individual is ready to return to work. Some patients may be required to carry a Holter monitor (about the size of a small portable tape recorder) around with them for twenty-four hours during a working day. This monitoring enables the physician to assess the heart's response to the stress of working. Monitoring also uncovers abnormal heart rhythms that might require treatment.

TABLE 3. *Approximate Metabolic Cost of Activities**

Self Care   Housework

ACTIVITY	METS	ACTIVITY	METS
Rest, supine	1	Hand sewing	1
Sitting	1	Sweeping floor	1.5
Standing, relaxed	1	Machine sewing	1.5
Eating	1	Polishing furniture	2
Conversation	1	Peeling potatoes	2.5
Dressing, undressing	2	Scrubbing, standing	2.5
Washing hands, face	2	Washing small	
Propulsion, wheelchair	2	clothes	2.5
Bedside commode	3	Kneading dough	2.5
Walking, 2.5 mph	3	Scrubbing floors	3
Showering	3.5	Cleaning windows	3
Using bedpan	4	Making beds	3
Walking downstairs	4.5	Ironing, standing	3.5
Walking, 3.5 mph	5.5	Mopping	3.5
Ambulation, braces		Wringing by hand	3.5
and crutches	6.5	Hanging wash	3.5
		Beating carpets	4

Occupational Activities

ACTIVITY	METS	ACTIVITY	METS
Watch repairing	1.5	Welding — moderate	
Armature winding	2	load	2.5
Cobbling	2.5	Bricklaying	3.5
Typing	2.5	Plastering	3.5
Bartending	2.5	Tractor plowing	3.5
Radio assembly	2.5	Wheelbarrowing	
Sewing at machine	2.5	115 lbs 2.5 mph	4

* 1 Met = amount of energy expended while sitting quietly in a chair.

Occupational Activities (cont.)

ACTIVITY	METS	ACTIVITY	METS
Painting, masonary	5	Planing	7.5
Paperhanging	5	Digging ditches	8
Horse plowing	5	Carrying 80 lbs	8
Carpentry	5	Tending furnace	8.5
Binding sheaves	5.5	Shoveling 10/min	
Shoveling light earth	6	(14 lbs)	9
Mowing lawn by		Shoveling 10/min	
hand	6.5–7	(16 lbs)	10+
Felling tree	6.5	Ascending stairs —	
Shoveling 10/min		22 lb load	
(10 lbs)	7	54'/min	13.5
Ascending stairs —			
17 lb load 27'/min	7.5		

Recreational and Outdoor Activities

ACTIVITY	METS	ACTIVITY	METS
Playing cards	1.5	Bowling	3
Painting, sitting	1.5	Cycling, 5.5 mph	3.5
Playing piano	2	Golfing	4
Driving car	2	Swimming, 20 yd/min	4
Riding lawnmower	2.5	Archery	4
Canoeing, 2.5 mph	2.5	Sailing — small boat	4
Horseback riding, slow	2.5	Fly fishing — standing	4
Volleyball	2.5	Badminton — doubles	4
Flying	3	Pushing light power	
Motorcycling	3	mower	4
Billiards	3	Energetic musician	4
Skeet	3	Rowing — leisurely	4
Shuffleboard	3	Dancing — foxtrot	5
Light woodworking	3	Gardening	5
Powerboat driving	3	Table tennis	5

ACTIVITY	METS	ACTIVITY	METS
Raking leaves	5	Mountain climbing	8
Tennis — doubles	5	Ice hockey	8
Hoeing	5	Canoeing (5 mph)	8
Sexual relations — conjugal	5	Touch football	8
		Paddleball	8
Stream fishing — walking in waders	6	Running (5 mph)	9
Trotting horse	6.5	Cycling (13 mph)	9
Ice or roller skating	7	Ski touring (4 mph) (loose snow)	9
Badminton — competitive	7	Squash racquets (social)	9
Tennis singles	7	Handball — social	9
Splitting wood	7	Fencing	9
Snow shoveling	7	Basketball (vigorous)	9
Hand lawn mowing	7	Running: 6 mph	10
Water skiing	7	7 mph	11.5
Folk (square) dancing	7	8 mph	13.5
Light downhill skiing	7	9 mph	15
Ski touring (2.5 mph) (loose snow)	7	10 mph	17
Jogging (5 mph)	8	Ski touring (5+ mph) (loose snow)	10+
Cycling (12 mph)	8		
Horseback (gallop)	8	Handball (competitive)	10+
Vigorous downhill skiing	8	Squash (competitive)	10+
Basketball	8		

Certain activities place excessive demands on the heart and should be avoided. Listed below are a number of situations that the heart attack patient should avoid.

1. Walking or other forms of exercise in very cold or very hot and humid weather.
2. Walking or other forms of exercise when tired or emotionally stressed.
3. Walking or other forms of exercise immediately after eating or drinking alcoholic beverages.
4. Exercise that requires straining such as lifting, pushing, or pulling heavy objects, or trying to open a stuck window or jar lid.
5. Straining when having a bowel movement.
6. Working with your arms above shoulder level. Try to rearrange drawers and cabinets so that things commonly used are at or below waist level.

Every patient is different with respect to how quickly activity can be resumed after myocardial infarction. Some patients may be candidates for *supervised* physical conditioning or training. A program of strenuous exercise should only be prescribed by a physician, and it should only be carried out under medical supervision.

Most physicians request their patients to return for a checkup four to six weeks after the heart attack. Further visits generally occur at two to four monthly intervals for one to two years and then at four to six monthly intervals thereafter.

12.
Sexual Activity after a Myocardial Infarction

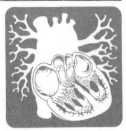

Maintaining normal sexual relations is important for an individual's sense of well-being. Ceasing sexual relations after a heart attack may disturb a previously harmonious relationship and bring psychological stress to bear on the patient and his/her partner. Moreover, the fact is that the amount of physical exertion required for normal sexual relations can almost always be tolerated by the patient without endangering his/her heart. Physicians' advice varies somewhat in the timing of resumption of sexual relations after a heart attack. In general, however, sexual intercourse may be resumed three to eight weeks following a myocardial infarction.

Many persons who have had a heart attack fear that sexual intercourse is life-threatening. Studies show this is rarely true. Sexual relations with a spouse or usual partner are about as strenuous as briskly climbing two flights of stairs. Some medical authorities believe that sexual intercourse with a new or unaccustomed partner demands more work from the heart and hence may be dangerous. Of course, responses vary among individuals, but certain suggestions are in order.

1. It is best to avoid having intercourse:
   a) immediately after a large meal
   b) for three hours after drinking alcohol
   c) in extremely hot or cold temperatures
   d) just before or after strenuous activity
   e) if you are feeling anger or resentment
   f) when you are very fatigued

2. Patients who experience angina during intercourse may obtain relief from this symptom by taking a nitroglycerin tablet in advance.

3. It is a good idea to allow ample time for "warm up" (foreplay), remembering that the patient and his/her partner have been apart for a while.

4. Consider just being intimate without orgasm or climax the first few times together — especially if either partner feels uneasy about resuming intercourse.

5. Suggested positions for intercourse that seem to require less energy are a) side-lying (Figure 8), b) "person-on-top-of-person" with the patient's partner on top (Figure 9), c) sitting in an armless chair facing each other. If it is difficult to change from an accustomed position, however, return to what is most familiar.

If you should experience any of the following, reconsider your approach to sexual activity and try progressing at a slower pace:

1. Rapid heart rate and/or rapid breathing lasting 20 to 30 minutes after intercourse.

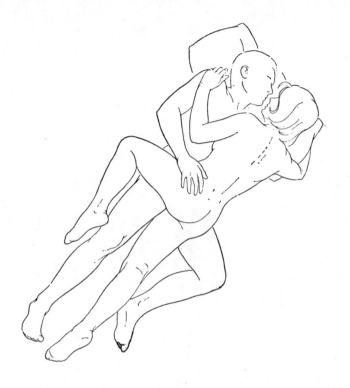

FIGURE 8. Lateral (Side) Intercourse Position

Couples frequently find it easier to start with the female superior intercourse position (Figure 9) and slide into the lateral intercourse position. Beginning with the female superior position, the woman leans forward against the man's chest while stretching out one leg behind her as noted in the drawing. The woman slides her body slightly toward the side of the man's bent knee. In this manner, the woman can have both knees touching the bed for traction. She is the active partner. This position is recommended when the male partner has suffered a heart attack.

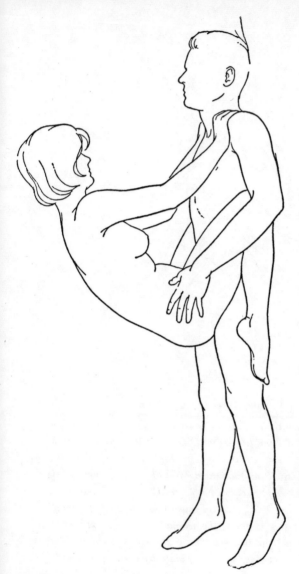

FIGURE 9. Female Superior (On Top) Intercourse Position

The female is the active partner. This intercourse position is recommended when the male partner has suffered a heart attack.

2. Chest pain during or after intercourse.
3. Sleeplessness or extreme fatigue on the day following intercourse.

Ultimately, the patient should be able to return to his/her previous level of sexual activity. Physicians are usually willing to discuss sexual matters with their patients, and the latter should not hesitate to ask the doctor for guidance.

Psychological Impact of a
Myocardial Infarction

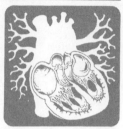

Patients who suffer a myocardial infarction frequently worry about two things: 1) the immediate threat to their life and 2) the long-term threat that their heart disease will significantly alter their life-style and livelihood. People commonly react to the threat of death by developing anxiety. It is also common to react to anticipated changes in a way of living by becoming depressed. Anxiety usually occurs during the first few days in the coronary care unit, while depression comes on a few days later and remains for a longer period of time. Anxiety is relieved once the patient discovers that he/she will, in fact, survive the heart attack. Depression is not so easily relieved in the hospital because many patients expect that there will be significant changes in their life-style after they return home. Thus, recovery from a heart attack involves reducing anxiety and depression.

Depression can be very hard to detect, since people are often unaware that they are depressed. Persons who suffer a heart attack are often only aware of a general feeling of weakness or uneasiness. Some patients find that the tranquilizers given them in the hospital result in a "blue feeling" as well as amnesia (loss of memory) for the earlier parts of the hospital stay. Other patients do not like to take sedatives or tranquilizers because they are afraid of becoming addicted to these drugs. This fear is unfounded; patients who use these drugs for the anxiety and depression that accompany a heart attack rarely, if ever, become addicted.

The best medicine for the anxiety and depression that accompany a heart attack is a frank discussion with a nurse and/or physician. Such discussions usually help the patient to appraise the situation realistically. Indeed, most patients can realistically expect to return to their jobs, leisure activities, and sexual relations. Time is required, however, for most patients to come to grips with their fears and to realize that the changes in their lives will not be as bad as anticipated.

It is not uncommon for depression to become worse after the patient's homecoming. Again, the patient is often not aware of this depression and feels it only as weakness, fatigue, or a sense of dependency. These symptoms may be particularly distressing since many individuals believe them to be signs of permanent cardiac disability. Besides depression, the prolonged period of bed rest that occurs during the recovery phase from a heart attack can also contribute to fatigue and weakness. It is important not to overreact to these symptoms, since, in most cases, they gradually fade as life returns to normal. Again, frank discussions with family, friends, and health professionals can improve the patient's well-being by producing a realistic appraisal of the situation. In most cases, health professionals will be able to reassure the patient about eventual return to most, if not all, forms of activity.

Two other psychological problems can bother the heart attack patient after discharge from the hospital. The individual may notice various kinds of chest discomfort. The normal stresses of daily life produce fleeting, minor chest aches, arising from small irritations of the rib joints and chest muscles. The patient is often acutely aware of any chest sensation, and these small chest pains may cause considerable anxiety. The fleeting nature of these harmless discomforts and their relation to arm, shoulder, and back exercise usually help to distinguish such pains from angina pectoris. As time passes, the heart attack patient learns to ignore minor chest wall aches and pains.

Patients who have had a protracted and complicated hospital course may develop separation anxiety upon discharge from the security of the hospital. This is a normal feeling after a prolonged hospital stay. Such anxieties gradually recede as the patient gains strength and confidence during rehabilitation from myocardial infarction.

Medications can help to relieve anxiety and depression, and many physicians prescribe such medicines for the first few weeks following a heart attack.

Listed below are a number of situations and feelings that may occur during the recovery phase. A few helpful suggestions for overcoming these situations are included.

1. Feelings of anxiety or depression are normal following a heart attack. The realization that a heart attack is a serious disease brings these feelings on. Becoming informed through reading can help relieve anxiety and depression. Friendly discussions with family, friends, and health professionals can also help relieve these feelings.

2. Boredom is very common following a heart attack because of enforced inactivity and because of the number of restrictions placed on the patient during the early phases of recovery. Try to choose activities that are varied and relaxing, and plan a number of different ones for each day. Reading and handicrafts are frequently good cures for boredom. This problem frequently fades away as the patient's activity increases.

3. Overprotection by one's family and friends can be a problem. It is important to be patient with family members since they also have to make an adjustment to the expected modifications in the patient's lifestyle. Friends who have had a heart attack may be helpful in this regard.

Rarely, some individuals are unable to overcome feelings of depression or anxiety following a myocardial infarction. In such cases, professional counselling from the physician or from a psychiatrist is helpful. Patients who find that they cannot tolerate a decrease in the stressful features of their life-style (for example, competition at work) may also benefit from psychiatric counselling.

Psychological Impact of Myocardial Infarction on the Patient's Family

Psychological adjustments to an individual's new status after a heart attack must be made by members of the family, just as the individual must adjust. The first weeks after the patient's homecoming can be particularly trying. Because of the psychological stresses alluded to earlier, individuals who have suffered a myocardial infarction can be difficult to live with. Family members may be afraid to refuse any request made by the patient for fear of precipitating another heart attack. In addition, family members may feel guilty of having caused the heart attack in the first place. The patient may use such feelings to manipulate family members to perform desired tasks. On the other hand, family members may be overprotective, refusing to include the individual in family problem-solving.

These vexations can make family life difficult in the immediate post–myocardial infarction period. There is no panacea for such difficulties. Open, frank communication of one's feelings would seem to be the best route to take. The passage of time and frequent discussions of problems should help to eliminate the psychological difficulties that family members face. Of course, family members may also benefit from discussions with the physician or with health professionals.

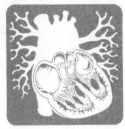

Patients who have suffered a heart attack may find themselves confronted with a confusing array of prescribed medications. This chapter explains the rationale behind the use of each of these agents. Drugs usually have two names: a generic, or chemical, name, and a brand, or trade, name. A drug may be manufactured by several different companies and hence appear under several brand names although it still has only one chemical name. It cannot be stressed enough that patients should take only those drugs prescribed specifically for them by a physician. Even if a friend or relative seems to have a similar or related heart condition, it can be extremely dangerous to "try" this person's medications (see General Rules for Taking Medications at end of chapter).

Some medications are prescribed for weeks to months after a heart attack, while other drugs will be taken for the rest of the patient's life. A number of different medications may be prescribed in combination, and frequent adjustments in the dosage of each medication may be required. It is a good idea for the patient to memorize drug names and dosages. Most drugs have multiple effects, some desired and some undesired. Undesired effects are known as side effects. On occasion, these side effects can be so troublesome that the medication must be discontinued.

Drugs That Strengthen the Heartbeat (Digitalis Preparations)

A number of different, but related, drugs extracted from the foxglove plant are used to strengthen and regulate the heart's contraction, or beat. Such drugs are usually used when heart failure, or poor pumping performance, appears. Digitalis is the generic name of the foxglove plant, and consequently all drugs derived from the plant are commonly referred to as "digitalis." The most commonly used form of digitalis is called digoxin (Lanoxin). A form less commonly employed is known as digitoxin.

Drugs in the digitalis family may cause significant side-effects when an excessive amount is taken. Side effects include: decreased appetite, nausea, palpitations (abnormal heart rhythm), nightmares, unusual fatigue, or visual disturbances.

Drugs That Reduce the Amount of Water Retained in the Body (Diuretics)

Patients with heart failure have a tendency to retain liquid in their bodies. This may manifest itself as shortness of breath or as swelling of the ankles. Such excess liquid can be removed from the body by means of a diuretic, a drug that increases the volume of urine produced by the patient. Excess body fluid can be eliminated by increasing the amount of urine excreted from the body. Many diuretics are available; the most commonly used ones include furosemide (Lasix), ethacrynic acid (Edecrin), chlorothiazide (Diuril), hydrochlorothiazide (HydroDiuril, Esidrix), triamterene (Dyrenium), spironolactone (Aldactone), and chlorthalidone (Hygroton).

Most diuretics result in a loss of the mineral potassium from the body. Consequently, many physicians prescribe a diet rich in potassium, and potassium-containing solutions (K-Lyte, Klorvess, Kay Ciel Elixer, and Slow-K) for patients on diuretics, to ensure that the body does not become depleted of potassium. Potassium depletion may cause muscle cramps, weakness, and palpitations or abnormal heart rhythm. Diuretics may cause the patient to become dehydrated and to feel weak and tired.

Drugs That Regulate the Heartbeat (Anti-arrhythmics)

Heart attack patients are prone to develop abnormal heart rhythms, or arrhythmias. There are many drugs that regulate the electrical activity of the heart and thereby the heart rhythm. Drugs in this class include quinidine, procainamide (Pronestyl), and diphenylhydantoin (Dilantin). Digoxin (Lanoxin), discussed earlier, and propranolol (Inderal), discussed later, have additional use in the control of heartbeat.

Drugs That Decrease the Work Load of the Heart
(Beta Blockers and Vasodilators)

The symptom of angina pectoris occurs when the work of the heart outstrips the ability of the coronary arteries to supply nourishing blood. Some medications are given to help reduce the work load imposed on the heart and hence reduce the frequency and severity of angina pectoris and/or heart failure. The work that the heart must perform can be reduced in a number of ways: by decreasing the blood pressure, heart rate, and the resistance that the blood vessels offer to the flowing blood. Drugs most commonly employed for this purpose include propranolol (Inderal), nitroglycerin (TNG), various forms of nitrates (Isordil, Sorbitrate, Cardilate), and hydralazine (Apresoline).

The side effects of propranolol include increased shortness of breath and stomach upset. Nitroglycerin, other forms of nitrates, and hydralazine can cause headaches and dizziness.

Drugs That Tranquilize or Relax (Tranquilizers)

Having a heart attack is an upsetting experience. For those individuals who require medication to reduce their anxiety, a large number of tranquilizing drugs exist. The tranquilizers most commonly used include diazepam (Valium), chlordiazepoxide hydrochloride (Librium), and meprobamate (Miltown).

Drugs That May Help Prevent Another Heart Attack
(Antihypertensive, Lipid-lowering Agents)

High blood pressure and elevated fat levels in the blood can hasten the development of coronary atherosclerosis. Consequently, individuals who suffer a heart attack should follow a program to make themselves less susceptible to another myocardial infarction. This is best accomplished by complying with their physician's advice and medication program aimed at reducing abnormal blood pressure or blood fat (cholesterol and/or triglycerides).

Medications that help to control blood pressure include many of the diuretics mentioned earlier. Other commonly employed antihypertensive (anti–high blood pressure) drugs include alpha methyldopa (Aldomet), hydralazine (Apresoline), clonidine (Catapres), reserpine, and guanethidine (Ismelin). A side effect common to all antihypertensive medications is dizziness experienced when the patient gets up from sitting or lying down. Such dizziness is due to a sudden, sharp drop in blood pressure. This symptom can usually be prevented if the patient sits or stands up slowly.

Elevated blood fat levels are usually controlled by a combination of diet and drugs. The diet prescribed may restrict fat and cholesterol intake in the manner described earlier (Chapter 9), or it may restrict other food substances such as starches and sugars. The diet prescribed depends on the kind of abnormal blood fat condition. There are five different ways in which abnormal blood fat can be expressed. Different combinations of

elevated blood cholesterol and/or triglycerides character-
ize each of these five conditions. Specific diets and medications can be effective in reducing the levels of cholesterol and triglyceride in such patients.

Medications commonly prescribed for elevated blood
fat include clofibrate (Atromid-S) and cholestyramine
(Questran). Digestive upset is the commonest side effect
of these two medications. (See also Appendix C, page
117.)

Blood-thinning Drugs (Anticoagulants)

Some physicians use blood-thinning medications
(anticoagulants) in treating patients who have heart
attacks. Such drugs decrease the ability of the blood to
clot or coagulate, but not all physicians believe that
blood thinners are beneficial, because of the additional
risk of bleeding complications with these drugs. Therefore, practices vary from doctor to doctor depending on
individual circumstances. Should the physician favor the
use of blood thinners, a number of different drugs can be
employed: heparin is given intravenously for three to ten
days after the myocardial infarction, followed by oral
warfarin (Coumadin, Dicumarol) for weeks to months.
Aspirin and/or dipyridamole (Persantine) are mild
blood thinners favored by some doctors.

Abnormal or excessive bleeding, from wounds or spon-
taneously, is the commonest side effect of blood thinners.
Any patient taking blood thinners should get careful
instructions from the physician concerning these medications before leaving the hospital.

Drugs Used to Treat Pericarditis (Irritation or Inflammation of the Membrane Surrounding the Heart)

As described earlier, pericarditis is an uncomfortable, but usually benign, complication of myocardial infarction. The pain of pericarditis is usually treated with aspirin or indomethacin (Indocin). This pain may develop weeks or even months after a heart attack and may require prolonged treatment.

Drugs Used to Reduce the Size of a Heart Attack

A number of investigators have been working to develop techniques that would reduce the extent of the damage from a heart attack that has already occurred. Reduction in the extent of damage of a heart attack means that less heart muscle is destroyed by a particular myocardial infarction.

A number of different drugs have been shown to be effective in reducing infarct size in animals and in human beings when given soon after the onset of myocardial infarction, although the work is still experimental. If further testing reveals that certain drugs can indeed reduce infarct size, then this form of treatment will become common in the future.

General Rules for Taking Medications

1. Try to stick to the dosage schedule prescribed by the doctor.

2. Speak to a physician (preferably one's own) before stopping any medication. This is particularly important with the drug propranalol (Inderal).

3. Medications are *only* for the patient for whom they were prescribed. Never try another patient's medication.

4. The idea that one pill is good and a second one twice as good is completely false and can be dangerous.

5. Many drugs can interact with each other inside the body. This interaction can result in dangerous side effects. Never take prescription or nonprescription medicines unless they have been cleared by a physician.

6. Side effects or allergic reactions to medications can and do occur. It is imperative that one contact a physician (preferably one's own) if side effects or allergic reactions to a medication are suspected.

Appendix A.
Questions for the Patient
at the Time of Discharge
from the Hospital

Patients and doctors form an alliance during the course of an illness. The purpose of this alliance is continuing improvement in the patient's condition. It is important that adequate communication occur between the patient and the doctor. This Appendix contains a number of questions for the heart attack patient. The patient should understand the answers to these questions and should clarify with the doctor any areas of confusion. Reproduced below is the discharge questionnaire for heart attack patients developed by Mrs. Jane Alexander, R.N., M.S.N., Cardiac Clinical Nurse at the Peter Bent Brigham Hospital, Boston.

Instructions for the Person Using This Questionnaire

Purpose: This questionnaire is designed to help determine what you know and what you need to learn regarding a heart attack. Please read and answer the questions that will help identify areas in which you need more knowledge. This questionnaire is *not* meant to test to see how *well* you do.

How To Complete The Form: Please read the questions and select the answer you feel to be true. If you are unsure of the answer, circle the selection marked "not sure." Questions that are answered incorrectly identify areas in which more information is needed. Take your time answering the questions.

NOTE: All questions refer to persons who have had a heart attack.

1. Which of the following statements about the heart is true?
   1) The heart is a muscle that requires a rich supply of oxygen to function.
   2) A natural pacemaker within the heart muscle causes the heart to beat.
   3) The heart acts as a pump for blood and is influenced by nerves and hormones.

   Answer
   a) 1, 2
   b) 2, 3
   c) 1, 3
   d) all of the above
   e) not sure

2. Angina pectoris is heart pain caused by a temporary condition of inadequate blood supply to the heart muscle. It usually:

a) lasts for hours.
b) lasts at least one to two minutes.
c) lasts over thirty minutes.
d) not sure

3. Persons with heart pain may describe it as any of the following *except:*
   a) squeezing or crushing in the center of the chest.
   b) heaviness under the breast bone.
   c) shooting pain across the ribs.
   d) not sure

4. A person comes to the hospital experiencing pain more severe than the usual angina. The discomfort is accompanied by sweating, nausea, and vomiting. It is determined at the hospital that the individual has experienced a heart attack. This means:
   a) There was no damage to the heart but the muscle was temporarily not getting enough blood.
   b) Some heart muscle was damaged due to lack of blood and will have to heal slowly, leaving a scar.
   c) Some heart muscle was damaged and will never heal completely, leaving a "soft spot" in the heart.
   d) Some heart muscle was damaged and will heal completely over time, leaving no trace.
   e) not sure

5. Complete healing of the heart following a heart attack takes approximately:
   a) one week
   b) six weeks
   c) six months
   d) not sure

6. On first entering the hospital, some patients are put on a heart monitor. The purpose of this is to:
   a) keep the heart beating.
   b) repair the heart electrically.
   c) detect changes in the electrical activity of the heart.
   d) not sure

7. A patient has a pacemaker inserted while in the hospital; the purpose of this is to:
   a) stimulate the heart to beat when it does not beat automatically.
   b) heal the damaged part of the heart.
   c) tell the nurses if the heart beat changes.
   d) not sure

8. A person who previously had a heart attack is watching an exciting television program at home and begins to have heart pain. This person should immediately:
   a) call the doctor and take a nitroglycerin tablet.
   b) take a nitroglycerin, turn off the TV and rest, sitting up.

c) take a nitroglycerin tablet and lie down.
d) call the doctor.
e) not sure

9. When a heart attack patient arrives home from the hospital, it is important to avoid:
   a) standing or walking.
   b) holding his/her breath and straining while lifting something.
   c) taking showers.
   d) not sure

10. Of the following activities, which is usually the last resumed by a heart attack patient at home?
    a) walking
    b) showering
    c) driving
    d) sexual intercourse
    e) not sure

11. A heart attack patient has been home from the hospital four weeks. Angina occurs with activity and is relieved by taking a nitroglycerin tablet and resting. The past few days the patient has begun having angina when resting and even during sleep. If the patient is scheduled to see the doctor again in three weeks, it is important to:
    a) go to the hospital immediately.
    b) call the doctor.
    c) just keep the regular appointment.
    d) not sure

12. If heart pain does not go away even after three nitroglycerin tablets taken five minutes apart, the person should:
    a) keep taking nitroglycerin tablets.
    b) come to the hospital.
    c) walk around to see if the pain goes away.
    d) not sure

13. While eating a meal at a cafeteria, one finds the following foods available. Which would be the healthiest choice?
    a) baked pork chops
    b) poached eggs and bacon
    c) broiled chicken
    d) not sure

14. At a friend's house alcoholic drinks are offered. It would be best to:
    a) refuse flatly.
    b) ask for several refills.
    c) accept the drink if you want it.
    d) not sure

15. A doctor has prescribed a low-salt diet for a patient. After preparing a meal without salt, the food may be seasoned with all the following except:
    a) pepper
    b) lemon juice
    c) vinegar
    d) soy sauce
    e) not sure

16. Doctors usually recommend that heart attack patients stop smoking and lose weight if overweight. If a patient who has stopped smoking gains five pounds, it is advisable to:
    a) resume smoking to cause weight loss.
    b) not resume smoking but attempt to avoid further weight gain.
    c) smoke only when feeling the urge to eat.
    d) not sure

17. When a person smokes cigarettes, which of the following is true?
    1) Blood pressure is increased.
    2) Damage to the lining of the arteries supplying blood to the heart muscle may occur.
    3) The person's work efficiency is increased.
    4) The ability of the blood to carry oxygen needed by the heart muscle is decreased.

    Answer
    a) 1, 2, 4
    b) 3
    c) all the above
    d) none of the above
    e) not sure

18. The doctor sends a patient home with several prescriptions for medicine. Concerning taking these medications, the patient should:
    a) not take them too long as one may become dependent on them.
    b) take extra medicine on bad days.

c) take a day off from medicines to let the body rest once a week.
d) check with the doctor before starting any new nonprescription drugs.
e) not sure

19. The doctor has advised a patient that he/she may now resume sexual relations. Which of the following would be recommended?
a) having relations after a hearty dinner.
b) having relations to help relax after an especially tiring day.
c) having the partner take a dominant or equal part in sexual activity.
d) having a cocktail before intercourse.
e) not sure

20. A married patient has been home from the hospital one week and finds that the relationship with his/her spouse is tense and awkward. Which of the following might be helpful to remember or do?
1) They have both had to cope with many stresses since the heart attack.
2) They both may feel uncertain about future job and home life.
3) Talking together about feelings may help reduce tension and prevent misunderstandings.
4) Avoiding discussion of conflicts between spouses always lessens tension.

Answer
a) 1

b) 1, 2, and 3
c) all the above
d) none of the above
e) not sure

21. A patient has returned to work or to homemaking. Which of the following would be helpful to do or remember?
1) Take regular rest periods throughout the day.
2) Spread activities throughout the day and avoid rushing.
3) If one feels very anxious or tense, leave the area temporarily to rest or relax.
4) Set limits on expectations of self.
5) Be really efficient to prove to one's employer or family that one is as good as new.

Answer
a) 1, 2, 5
b) 5 only
c) 1, 2, 3, 4
d) 3, 4
e) not sure

22. Mr. Smith and Mr. Jones work for the same company and have the same job as office manager. Which of the two men has a life-style and personality more commonly associated with heart attack?

Mr. Smith	*Mr. Jones*
works overtime often	works an 8-hour day
drinks 2–3 cups coffee daily	drinks 2–3 cups coffee daily

plans to be company president	enjoys being office manager
is 10 pounds over-weight	is 15 pounds over-weight
smokes 2 packs per day	does not smoke
is frequently dissatisfied with himself	feels he is doing well
rushes everywhere	takes his time doing tasks
skipped vacation last year	will take a two-week vacation

Answer
a) Mr. Smith
b) Mr. Jones
c) not sure

KEY

Question Number	Answer	Question Number	Answer
1.	d	12.	b
2.	b	13.	c
3.	c	14.	c
4.	b	15.	d
5.	b	16.	b
6.	c	17.	a
7.	a	18.	d
8.	b	19.	c
9.	b	20.	b
10.	c	21.	c
11.	b	22.	a

It is important that the patient understand the significance of a heart attack and the best route to recovery. Any of the above questions that seemed difficult or for which the wrong answer was selected should be reviewed with a doctor or nurse.

In addition, it is important that the patient understand:

1) Any limitations of activity after discharge.
2) The nature and schedule of discharge medications.
3) What to do should heart pain recur.

Any doubts in the patient's mind concerning these three areas should be thoroughly discussed with the doctor and/or nurse.

Appendix B.
Questions Commonly
Asked by Patients

Many questions arise in the mind of any patient following a heart attack or the development of the symptoms of angina pectoris. Unfortunately, all too often when the moment arrives to place these questions before the doctor, they are suddenly forgotten. Listed below are those most frequently asked by my patients who have coronary artery disease. The questions, with their answers, are listed by topic.

Causes of Coronary Artery Disease

Q.   What is coronary artery disease?

A.   Coronary artery disease is a process that involves a gradual deposition of fatty materials around the inner walls of the coronary arteries. Over a period of time, these deposits narrow and choke off the passageways of the coronary arteries.

Q. What factors increase the risk of developing coronary artery disease?

A. A number of factors have been shown to increase one's risk of developing coronary artery disease. Such factors include advanced age, cigarette smoking, high blood pressure, elevated fat substances in the blood (cholesterol and triglyceride), inactivity, obesity, and psychological stress.

Angina Pectoris and Myocardial Infarction

Q. What causes the discomfort of angina pectoris or myocardial infarction?

A. Lack of blood flow to heart muscle.

Q. Does any damage occur to the heart with episodes of angina pectoris?

A. No.

Q. Does any damage occur to the heart with a myocardial infarction?

A. Yes. With myocardial infarction, some of the heart muscle actually dies.

Q. Is angina pectoris or myocardial infarction always associated with discomfort in the chest?

A. No. Many individuals have discomfort only in their arms, neck, jaw, or back.

Q. What sort of discomfort is typical of angina pectoris?

A. Angina pectoris is characterized by a heaviness, burning, squeezing, tightening, or pressure-like discomfort in the middle of the chest, usually behind the breastbone. However, many individuals have discomfort in their arms, neck, jaw, and back.

Q. What should one do if an episode of angina pectoris is not relieved by rest and two nitroglycerin tablets under the tongue?

A. Have someone take you to the hospital emergency room.

Q. How soon after a nitroglycerin tablet dissolves under the tongue should the discomfort of angina pectoris begin to fade?

A. Within a few minutes.

Q. How soon should the episode of discomfort be completely gone?

A. Within five to fifteen minutes.

Q. What is the difference between the discomfort of angina pectoris and the discomfort of myocardial infarction?

A. The discomfort associated with angina pectoris is short-lived and usually disappears after a few minutes following rest and nitroglycerin therapy. The discomfort of myocardial infarction usually increases, is not relieved by nitroglycerin, and lasts for a considerable amount of time, usually in excess of thirty minutes. The discomfort of myocardial infarction is frequently associated with nausea, sweating, and light-headedness.

Q. What is a heart attack?

A. A heart attack is the death of a part of the heart muscle from insufficient nutrition by the blood.

Q. What causes a heart attack?

A. Narrowing of the coronary blood vessels, or coronary atherosclerosis, decreases the supply of nutritive blood to a part of the heart muscle, thus resulting in its death.

Q. What complications can occur in the heart because of a heart attack?

A. 1) Problems with the electrical system resulting in abnormal heart rhythms. 2) Increased heart muscle stiffness. 3) Heart failure. Complications 2 and 3 result in a "backup" of blood behind the heart.

Q. Can the complications of a heart attack be treated, and where is this best done?

A. Complications of a heart attack can be treated with a variety of medicines and procedures. This is best done in a coronary care unit.

Q. What kinds of abnormal electrical activity can occur in the heart following a heart attack and how can this problem be treated?

A. Following a myocardial infarction, one may develop abnormal fast or irregular heartbeat rhythms, or one may develop an electrical short circuit with very slow heart rhythms. These two irregularities are treated with medications and/or with an electrical pacemaker.

Q. What symptom is associated with heart failure after a myocardial infarction?

A. Shortness of breath is a very common symptom in patients who have heart failure.

Treatment

Q. What changes in life-style are required by the patient who suffers a heart attack?

A. Cessation of smoking, weight reduction, and decreased physical and emotional stress are beneficial to patients after a myocardial infarction. Many patients require medication to regulate the heartbeat, the blood pressure, or the blood cholesterol level.

Q. What is the purpose of the coronary care unit?

A. The coronary care unit provides a special protective environment for the treatment of patients who have suffered a heart attack.

Q. What is the purpose of the small paper or plastic electrodes that are placed on the chests of patients in the coronary care unit?

A. The electrodes help monitor the electrical activity of the heart. They enable the doctors and nurses in the coronary care unit to identify problems in the electrical activity of the heart and to treat these problems.

Q. Why do all patients in the coronary care unit have small needles or tubes placed in their veins?

A. These needles and tubes are placed in the veins of all patients in the coronary care unit in order to administer into the blood various medications necessary in the treatment of individuals with myocardial infarction.

Q. What medicines are frequently administered to relieve the discomfort associated with myocardial infarction?

A. Narcotics such as morphine or Demerol, and gases such as laughing gas.

Q. What is pericarditis and how is it treated?

A. Pericarditis is an irritation or inflammation of the membrane that surrounds the heart. Pericarditis often follows a heart attack, and it is treated with aspirin or indomethacin (Indocin).

Q. What are the commonest medications used to treat heart failure following a myocardial infarction?

A. Digitalis preparations, which strengthen the heartbeat, and diuretic preparations, which increase the amount of urine produced by the kidneys, are the two medications most commonly used to treat heart failure following a heart attack.

Q. Why is a pacemaker necessary?

A. Damage to the electrical system of the heart can result in a dangerous slowing of the heartbeat. A pacemaker ensures that the heart rate stays above a certain minimum number, for example, seventy beats per minute.

Q. What constitutes a pacemaker?

A. A pacemaker has two parts: a wire, one end of which is inserted into the heart, and a battery-powered pacemaker box, which is attached at the other end of the wire. When a pacemaker is inserted permanently, this box is placed under the skin.

Q. Are there any special precautions for pacemaker patients?

A. No; pacemaker patients may lead an active, normal life.

Q. Can atherosclerotic narrowings in coronary arteries be removed surgically?

A. No, such narrowings usually cannot be removed, but blood can be delivered to the heart muscle bypassing such areas of narrowing by means of the heart operation known as the coronary artery bypass.

Q. Should all patients who have a heart attack undergo coronary artery surgery?

A. Coronary artery surgery (coronary bypass grafting) is usually reserved for patients suffering with severe and/or incapacitating angina pectoris. Not all patients who have a heart attack develop angina pectoris, and hence not all patients who have a heart attack are candidates for coronary artery bypass.

Occasionally, patients with very severe coronary artery disease but only mild symptoms may require coronary artery surgery.

Q. Which symptom is best relieved by coronary artery surgery and which is not?

A. The symptom of angina pectoris is relieved in over 90 percent of cases by coronary artery surgery. Shortness of breath is usually not helped by this operation.

Q. What is the purpose of cardiac catheterization?

A. Cardiac catheterization helps to identify with precision abnormal areas in the heart chambers and arteries. It may assist the cardiologist in making a correct diagnosis or it may be used to help plan for cardiac surgery.

Diet

Q. What factors in the American diet contribute to the development of heart attacks?

A. Overeating and too much fat in the diet.

Q. What are some foods that are particularly high in cholesterol and/or saturated fat and should therefore be avoided?

A. Eggs, meats, dairy products with high butterfat content, chocolate, delicatessen meats, coconut, and cashew nuts.

Q. Is the use of alcohol forbidden for persons who have suffered a heart attack?

A. No; moderate usage of alcoholic beverages is allowed.

Activity, Psyche, and Sex

Q. Isn't it true that most patients become semi-invalids after a heart attack?

A. Definitely not. Most individuals who suffer a heart attack return to active, vigorous lives. Many myocardial infarction patients find themselves fully able to enjoy work, hobbies, sports, and sexual activity.

Q. What factors cause the recuperative phase after a heart attack to differ from person to person?

A. The size of the heart attack, the patient's age and recuperative powers, and the history of other illnesses all influence the rate of recovery.

Q. What happens to an individual's heart rate with exercise?

A. The heart, or pulse, rate increases with increasingly strenuous exercise.

Q. What level of heart rate is allowable in the early (3 to 6 weeks) and late (6 to 12 weeks) recuperative phase after myocardial infarction?

A. 100 to 110 beats/ minute: early phase
120 to 130 beats/ minute: late phase

Q. Do heart attack patients ever return to normal activity levels after their myocardial infarction?

A. Yes; most patients who suffer a myocardial infarction can eventually return to a full and normal life style.

Q. Is it uncommon for individuals to be anxious or depressed following a heart attack?

A. It is normal to be anxious or depressed following a heart attack.

Q. What is the best way to overcome one's anxiety or depression?

A. Frank discussions with friends, family, and health professionals usually help the patient to understand that the required changes in his/her life will not be drastic. The realization that one will return to job, leisure, and sexual activities helps relieve anxiety and depression.

Q. Are tranquilizing or antidepressant medications habit-forming when taken by patients following a heart attack?

A. No, these medications are not habit-forming when taken by patients specifically for anxiety or depression that occur following a heart attack.

Q. How soon after a myocardial infarction may the heart attack patient resume sexual relations?

A. In most cases, moderate sexual relations may be resumed immediately or shortly after discharge from the hospital.

Q. Is the "person-on-top-of-person" intercourse position the only one allowed for heart attack patients?

A. No; patients should employ whatever intercourse position feels most natural and comfortable. The "person-on-top-of-person" position requires less effort for the individual underneath, and hence it may be easier for the heart attack patient to employ this position.

Medicines are listed in alphabetical order. The first name is the generic or chemical name of the drug. Drug names (one or more) in parentheses following the generic name are brand names for that particular medication.

Allopurinol (Zyloprim) : This medication is used to prevent and treat gout. Gout is a disease in which excessive amounts of uric acid, a chemical produced by the body, accumulate in the joints and cause severe joint pain. Allopurinol helps to decrease the level of uric acid in the body. It is not uncommon for patients with coronary artery disease to have gout. Side effects of the drug include rashes, nausea, diarrhea, and drowsiness.

Aspirin: This commonly used medication has mild blood thinning (anticoagulant) properties (see *Dipyridamole*) .

Atropine sulfate: This drug blocks the effects of the vagus nerve on the heart. Since the vagus nerve controls slowing of the heart rate, blocking its action results in speeding of the heart rate. Thus, atropine is used to speed the heart rate when it becomes too slow. The drug is always given intravenously. Side effects include blurred vision, dry mouth, constipation, and difficulty urinating.

Chlordiazepoxide hydrochloride (Librium) : A mild tranquilizer. Side effects include drowsiness, dizziness.

Chlorothiazide (Diuril) : A medication that acts on the kidneys to increase urine flow (diuretic) and hence aids in removing excess fluid from the body. It is used to treat heart failure symptoms (shortness of breath, swelling of ankles or legs) and high blood pressure. The increased urine flow that accompanies ingestion of this drug can wash considerable amounts of the mineral potassium from the body. Therefore, it is common for physicians to prescribe potassium supplements for patients receiving diuretics. Side effects include nausea, dizziness, muscle aches or cramps, fatigue, and skin rashes.

Chlorthalidone (Hygroton) : A long-acting diuretic (see *Chlorothiazide*) .

Cholestyramine (Questran) : This drug lowers blood cholesterol levels (see *Clofibrate*) . Side effects include constipation, abdominal cramps, nausea, indigestion.

Clofibrate (Atromid-S) : This drug lowers blood fat levels (cholesterol, triglyceride) . It is expected that lowering of blood lipid (fat) levels decreases the rate of accumulation of atherosclerotic deposits in blood vessels. Side effects include nausea, loose stools, indigestion, muscle aches and cramps, and the risk of gallstones with long-term use. The possibility of more dangerous side effects is currently under study.

Clonidine hydrochloride (Catapres) : This medication lowers blood pressure (antihypertensive, see *Methyldopa*). Side effects include dry mouth and dizziness.

Diazepam (Valium) : A mild tranquilizer (see *Chlordiazepoxide hydrochloride*).

Digitoxin: A long-acting digitalis preparation (see *Digoxin*).

Digoxin (Lanoxin) : A drug that strengthens the heartbeat and thus helps to relieve the symptoms of heart failure (shortness of breath, ankle or leg swelling, fatigue). Digoxin is also used to control heart rate and to abolish abnormal heart rhythms (cardiac arrhythmias). Side effects include loss of appetite, nausea, visual disturbances, and nightmares.

Dioctyl sulfosuccinate (Colace, Surfak) : This medication softens stools and keeps bowel movements loose and easy to pass. It aids patients with coronary artery disease in avoiding potentially dangerous straining at stool. Side effects are limited to excessive loosening of stools.

Diphenylhydantoin (Dilantin) : This drug is used to control abnormal heart rhythms that originate in the ventricles (ventricular arrhythmias). The drug is more often used to control seizures in patients with epilepsy. Side effects include skin rashes, excessive growth of gum tissue, dizziness, loss of balance, nausea, and anemia.

Dipyridamole (Persantine) : This medication is a mild blood thinner (anticoagulant). It is often used in combination with warfarin, aspirin, or both to prevent blood clot formation within the cardiovascular system. Side effects include dizziness, headache, nausea, and skin rash.

Dopamine (Intropin) : This drug increases the strength of the heartbeat and also raises the blood pressure. It is used to treat the more severe manifestations of left ventricular failure. The drug is always given intravenously. Side effects include nausea, headache, and palpitations.

Epinephrine (Adrenalin) : This drug increases the strength of the heartbeat and also raises the blood pressure (see *Dopamine*).

Erythrityl tetranitrate (Cardilate) : This medication is a long-acting form of nitroglycerin (see *Nitroglycerin*).

Ethacrynic acid (Edecrin) : A potent diuretic (see *Chlorothiazide*).

Flurazepam hydrochloride (Dalmane) : A mild sleep medicine (sedative). Side effects include excessive and prolonged drowsiness and dizziness.

Furosemide (Lasix) : A potent diuretic (see *Chlorothiazide*).

Guanethidine (Ismelin) : This medication lowers blood pressure (antihypertensive, see *Methyldopa*). Side effects include skin rashes and dizziness.

Heparin: This drug is a bloodthinner (anticoagulant). It prevents blood clot formation in the heart, veins, and arteries. It is used to prevent or treat episodes of blood clot formation within the cardiovascular system. Side effects include excessive bleeding from small injuries and internal bleeding. Frequent blood tests are performed when heparin is administered, in order to regulate the dose of the drug.

Hydralazine hydrochloride (Apresoline): This medication lowers blood pressure (antihypertensive, see *Methyldopa*). Side effects include skin rashes, anemia, dizziness, and palpitations.

Hydrochlorothiazide (HydroDiuril, Esidrix): A diuretic (see *Chlorothiazide*).

Indomethacin (Indocin): This drug helps to decrease inflammation and irritation (anti-inflammatory). It is used to treat the discomfort of pericarditis (inflammation of the lining surrounding the heart), which can occur after myocardial infarction. Side effects include indigestion, blurred vision, anemia, and skin rashes.

Isoproterenol (Isuprel): This drug increases the strength of the heartbeat. It can also raise blood pressure under certain circumstances. Isoproterenol is not employed very frequently in the coronary care unit, but it is used commonly after cardiac surgery (see *Dopamine*).

Isosorbide dinitrate (Isordil, Sorbitrate): This medication is a long-acting form of nitroglycerin (see *Nitroglycerin*).

Levarterenol, norepinephrine (Levophed): This drug raises the blood pressure. It increases the vigor of heart contraction to a minor degree (see *Dopamine*).

Lidocaine: This drug helps to control abnormal heart rhythms originating in the ventricles (ventricular arrhythmias). The drug can only be administered intravenously. Side effects include confusion and, rarely, convulsions.

Meperidine hydrochloride (Demerol): A narcotic synthesized in the laboratory (see *Morphine*).

Methyldopa (Aldomet): This medication lowers blood pressure (antihypertensive). It is used to treat patients with high blood pressure (hypertension). Side effects include skin rashes, anemia, and dizziness.

Morphine: A narcotic derived from the opium poppy. It is a very effective pain-killer. Moreover, it can decrease the symptom of shortness of breath. Side effects include nausea, constipation, difficulty urinating, and drowsiness.

Nitroglycerin: This drug is one of the most important parts of the therapeutic program for patients with coronary artery disease. The medication helps to dilate (open) small blood vessels in the heart as well as in the rest of the body. It can lower blood pressure, and in this manner the drug decreases the work of the heart. Nitroglycerin can decrease the symptoms of angina pectoris and shortness of breath. Side effects include headache, palpitations, and dizziness. Appendix D lists some guidelines for the proper use of nitroglycerin.

Pentaerythritol tetranitrate (Peritrate) : This medication is a long-acting form of nitroglycerin (see *Nitroglycerin*).

Potassium replacements (Kay Ciel Elixer, Klorvess, Slow-K, K-Lyte) : Diuretic medications (fluid pills) cause the body to lose the mineral potassium. This mineral is essential for normal nerve, muscle, and heart function. Potassium replacements are therefore frequently given to patients with heart disease who are taking diuretics. Side effects are usually limited to indigestion.

Prazosin hydrochloride (Minipress) : This medication lowers blood pressure (antihypertensive, see *Methyldopa*). Side effects include dizziness, headache, fatigue, and nausea.

Probenecid (Benemid) : This medication is used to treat patients with gout (see *Allopurinol*).

Procainamide (Pronestyl) : A drug used to control abnormal heart rhythms (anti-arrhythmic). Pronestyl is usually used to combat abnormal heart rhythms from the lower heart chambers (ventricular arrhythmias). Side effects include skin rashes, fevers, anemia, nausea, diarrhea, and dizziness.

Propranolol (Inderal) : This drug has three important uses: 1) It is effective in controlling both atrial and ventricular arrhythmias (abnormal heart rhythms), 2) It decreases blood pressure and can therefore be used to control high blood pressure, 3) It slows the heartbeat and thereby decreases the work of the heart. This action of propranolol makes it particularly effective in decreasing the frequency of attacks of angina pectoris. Side effects include skin rashes, diarrhea, shortness of breath, and loss of hair.

Quinidine, quinidine sulfate (Quinaglute) : A drug used to control abnormal heart rhythms (anti-arrhythmic). Quinidine can be used to control abnormal heart beats from the upper heart chambers (atrial arrhythmias) or the lower heart chambers (ventricular arrhythmias). Side effects include nausea, diarrhea, and skin rashes.

Reserpine (Serpasil) : This medication lowers blood pressure (antihypertensive, see *Methyldopa*). Side effects include indigestion, dizziness, and depression.

Spironolactone (Aldactone) : A mild diuretic that does not wash the mineral potassium from the body (see *Chlorothiazide*).

Triamterene (Dyrenium) : A mild diuretic that does not wash the mineral potassium from the body (see *Chlorothiazide*).

Warfarin (Coumadin, Dicumarol) : This drug is a blood thinner (anticoagulant). Frequent blood tests are performed to help regulate the dose of the drug (see *Heparin*).

Appendix D.
Guidelines for the Proper Use of Nitroglycerin*

1. Nitroglycerin is one of the best available medications for the relief of chest discomfort (angina pectoris) resulting from inadequate blood flow to the heart muscle.

2. Nitroglycerin comes in small tablets. When needed, one nitroglycerin tablet is placed under the tongue and allowed to dissolve. This takes about 20 to 30 seconds.

3. Nitroglycerin can also be chewed with good effect. However, it should not be swallowed since it is absorbed directly into the bloodstream from the floor of the mouth.

4. The action of nitroglycerin is prompt, and relief of chest discomfort is generally obtained within one or two minutes.

* Modified from "Guidelines for the Proper Use of Nitroglycerin," a patient handout prepared and employed at the Peter Bent Brigham Hospital, Boston, by Dr. Howard R. Horn.

5. Nitroglycerin provokes a minor tingling or stinging sensation in the mouth, and this indicates that the pill has not lost its strength.

6. One of the first effects one experiences with nitroglycerin is a fullness, a warm sensation, or a throbbing in the head. This indicates that nitroglycerin is dilating blood vessels and improving circulation in the head as well as in the heart.

7. Nitroglycerin should be used immediately and without hesitation at the first hint of chest discomfort.

8. There are many discomforts or pains in the chest area that do not arise from the heart; nitroglycerin will not relieve these pains.

9. Nitroglycerin is not habit forming. It is not a narcotic or a painkiller. One can take nitroglycerin many times a day. No matter how often one uses nitroglycerin, it will always continue to work.

10. Nitroglycerin should be kept in one's pocket at all times.

11. Nitroglycerin tablets lose their effectiveness within a few months after a bottle is unsealed. In order to retain maximum potency, keep the tablets in the original glass bottle with the cotton removed and the metal top securely screwed on.

12. When taking nitroglycerin, it helps to be seated or standing. Do not lie down if it can be avoided.

13. If chest discomfort wakes one from sleep, be sure to keep nitroglycerin on the bedside night table. Be sure to sit up while taking it.

14. If a single nitroglycerin tablet does not relieve the chest discomfort within two to three minutes, take a second one; if discomfort is constant or if the relief is transient and then recurs, take a third pill; if, however, the discomfort is not completely controlled or continues to recur, the patient should be driven to the nearest hospital emergency ward for further attention. Do not waste valuable time on the telephone.

15. When chest discomfort is promptly relieved by nitroglycerin, it is unnecessary to interrupt activity. A moderate decrease in the pace of activity is advisable, however.

16. Nitroglycerin is most helpful when taken at the onset of discomfort rather than after discomfort has been present for several minutes.

17. If one knows that a certain activity, exertion, or excitement will bring on an anginal episode, angina can be prevented by taking a nitroglycerin tablet before the discomfort emerges. This is the wisest way to take nitroglycerin — in anticipation of discomfort.

18. Angina pectoris is especially likely to occur with:
    a) brisk walking outside on a cold day.
    b) walking or other exertion after a heavy meal.
    c) working under the time pressures of a deadline.
    d) performing public speaking.
    e) during sexual intercourse.

    If the patient has angina at these times, one or more nitroglycerin tablets before such events or activities should prevent or ease the episode.

Appendix E.
Guide to Tests Performed on Patients with Coronary Artery Disease

Numerous technical advances of the last twenty years enable physicians to obtain a great deal of information about the structure and function of the heart. Listed below in alphabetical order are the diagnostic procedures most commonly performed on patients who have coronary artery disease. These tests supply information that physicians use to regulate various forms of therapy.

Blood Tests — Numerous blood tests are performed on the patient with myocardial infarction. Enzymes (chemicals used by the heart muscle to function normally) are released from the damaged heart tissue into the bloodstream. Abnormal levels of the enzymes (CPK, SGOT, LDH) can be measured in a blood sample, thereby demonstrating that heart muscle damage has occurred. Various blood tests also measure the amount of a drug present in the body. These help the physician to give the patient the correct amount of a particular drug.

Cardiac Catheterization — This test has already been discussed in Chapter 7. It is an invasive procedure, that is, the skin is broken and instruments are introduced into the body. All invasive tests involve some discomfort (despite the use of anesthetics) and some (usually minimal) risk to the patient.

There are a number of different measurements that can be made during cardiac catheterization. Not all are made with every catheterization. The procedure is tailored to each patient since the doctor requires different diagnostic information for different patients. The various possible features of a cardiac catheterization include: measurements of heart pressures and blood flow (hemodynamics), x-ray photos or movies of the inside of the heart and its blood vessels (angiography), and determinations of the integrity of the electrical conduction network of the heart (bundle-of-His recordings).

Cardiac Graphics (*phonocardiogram, apexcardiogram, carotid pulse tracing, jugular venous pulse tracing*) — Recordings are made of the heart sounds and the shape of the carotid artery pulse (in the neck), the jugular vein pulse (also in the neck), and the impulse made when the tip of the heart strikes the inside of the chest wall (apexcardiogram). These tests provide information about the function of the heart and its valves. The test is noninvasive (the skin is not broken) and painless.

Cardiac Series — These are a series of four x-ray pictures of the heart and lungs taken from four different angles. Important information about enlarged or otherwise abnormal heart chambers can be obtained from the cardiac series. This is a noninvasive test (the skin is not broken) and is thus painless.

Chest X-ray — An x-ray picture of the chest shows the heart and lungs. Such an x-ray picture yields important information about the effect of a myocardial infarction on the functional state of the heart.

Echocardiogram — An image of parts of the heart chambers, valves and pericardium is obtained by means of an electronic machine that bounces high frequency sound waves (sonar) off various parts of the heart. A very exact and detailed picture of the heart structures can be obtained with this device. The test is performed noninvasively (without having to break the skin) and is therefore painless.

Electrocardiogram — A recording of the electrical activity of the heart. Each individual heart cell has electrical activity. The sum of the electrical activity of all heart cells is recorded by the electrocardiogram. This test measures many facets of cardiac function: the quantity of functioning heart muscle, areas of damaged heart muscle, and any abnormality in heart rhythm. The test is noninvasive (the skin is not broken) and is therefore painless.

Hemodynamic Monitoring — During the early phases of a heart attack, it may be necessary to obtain measurements from the inside of the heart. These measurements help to guide therapy during the early, critical phase following myocardial infarction. Two types of catheter (small plastic tube) may be inserted into the body to make these measurements. A pulmonary artery catheter is positioned in the blood vessel that leaves the right side of the heart. Measurements made with this catheter help to determine the degree of heart failure present and the amount of blood filling the left ventricular chamber. An arterial catheter is placed in an arm or leg artery. Blood pressure measurements and samples of blood for oxygen content are obtained using this catheter.

Not all heart attack patients require such catheters. Hemodynamic monitoring is only used as a guide to therapy for patients with large infarctions, heart failure, or other complications.

Holter Monitor — This device is a small, portable, tape recorder connected to several electrocardiographic paper electrodes taped to the skin. The system records all electrical activity of the heart during a twelve- to twenty-four-hour period. In this manner infrequent arrhythmias (abnormal heartbeats) can be detected. This test is noninvasive (the skin is not broken) and is therefore painless.

Radioisotope Studies — A number of hospital tests involve the injection of radioactive chemicals into the body. These compounds migrate into specific organs and reveal abnormal areas within these organs. Three types of radioisotope study can be performed in patients with acute myocardial infarction:

1. Infarction imaging — Certain radioactive compounds migrate into damaged heart muscle. A ma-

chine that detects radioactivity (scintillation detector) produces a photograph of the heart that shows areas of radioisotope concentration. If such areas are present, this is strong evidence that heart muscle damage has occurred.

2. Radioisotope ventriculogram — This study involves the labeling of blood cells with a radioactive compound. A radiation detector is positioned over the heart, and with the help of a computer, one obtains several different measurements of the efficiency of heart function. This test helps the physician decide how much damage has been done to the heart and how much residual heart function exists.

3. Lung scan — In this test, a radioactive compound is injected into the circulation of the lungs. Areas of the lungs that have blood clots in them (an abnormal condition known as pulmonary embolism) are revealed by this test. Patients who have had heart attacks occasionally have episodes during which blood clots form in the legs and migrate to the lungs, disturbing heart and lung function. Blood thinners, or anticoagulants, are prescribed when this occurs.

Vectorcardiogram — A three-dimensional recording of the electrical activity of the heart. In some instances it supplies more information than a routine electrocardiogram (see *Electrocardiogram*) about areas of damaged heart muscle. This test is noninvasive (the skin is not broken) and is therefore painless.

Glossary

Angina pectoris. A discomfort in the chest that arises from a deficiency of blood reaching heart muscle.

Angiogram. An x-ray study in which dye is injected through small plastic tubes into the heart or blood vessels. The x-ray photos or movies that are made during injection of this dye reveal abnormalities in the heart or blood vessels.

Apexcardiogram. A painless diagnostic test that helps to measure heart function (see *Appendix E, Cardiac Graphics*).

Arrhythmias. Abnormal heartbeats, usually irregular, which often occur during a heart attack. Frequently medical treatment is necessary to restore heartbeats to their normal pattern.

Artery. A blood vessel that carries nourishing, oxygen-rich blood from the heart to the other organs of the body.

Atherosclerosis. A process in which fatty substances in the blood are deposited within the walls of blood vessels. These fatty deposits narrow the blood vessels and decrease the amount of blood that flows through these vessels. Also called arteriosclerosis.

Atrium. A heart chamber that primes or optimally fills the pumping chamber (ventricle). Also called an auricle.

Balloon pump. This device (in full called the intra-aortic balloon counterpulsation pump) is used to support the hearts of patients who have suffered a large complicated myocardial infarction (see *Chapter 5*).

Blood pressure. Pressure generated within the circulatory system by the interaction of the heart pumping blood and the resistance of the blood vessels to this pumped blood. There are two parts to a blood pressure measurement: the systolic blood pressure is the highest number, and it occurs when the left ventricle is pumping; the diastolic blood pressure is the lower number, and it occurs when the heart is filling.

Bradycardia. An abnormally slow heart rate.

Carbon monoxide. A poisonous gas inhaled during smoking of cigarettes. Carbon monoxide combines with elements in the blood and prevents them from carrying their normal amount of oxygen.

Cardiac catheterization. A diagnostic test performed by specially trained cardiologists (see *Chapter 7*).

Cardiac series. A series of four x-ray views of the heart and lungs (see *Appendix E, Cardiac Series*).

Cardioversion. The delivery of electric shock to the heart to stop cardiac arrhythmias (abnormal heartbeat).

Cardioverter. A device for delivering electric shock to the heart to stop cardiac arrhythmias.

Carotid pulse tracing. A painless diagnostic test used to measure heart function (see *App. E, Cardiac Graphics*).

Catheter. A tube or wire placed into the heart or the blood vessels leading to or from the heart. Catheters have different functions: obtaining blood samples from the heart chambers and measuring electrical activity in different heart chambers.

Cholesterol. A fatty substance, essential to life, that is a normal constituent of blood. Elevated levels of blood cholesterol predispose individuals to atherosclerosis and myocardial infarction.

Clot. A gelatinous clump of blood that can form within a blood vessel and thereby hinder the flow of blood.

Collateral blood vessels. Reserve blood vessels, present from birth, that open as the usually employed blood vessels become narrowed by atherosclerotic deposits.

Congestive heart failure (congestion). See *Heart failure.*

Coronary artery. A blood vessel that supplies the heart with nourishing blood. There are three major coronary arteries that supply the heart in human beings.

Coronary artery bypass graft. A surgical procedure that introduces new blood into the heart. An expendable vein is removed from the leg and is inserted into the heart beyond areas of atherosclerotic narrowing.

Coronary artery disease. The commonest lethal disease in the United States today. This disease results from narrowings in the coronary arteries from atherosclerotic deposits that build up there. These narrowings eventually cause myocardial infarction. The coronary arteries seem to be particularly predisposed to developing atherosclerotic narrowings.

CPK. An enzyme present in heart muscle that is released into the bloodstream when heart muscle becomes damaged. Measurement of this enzyme in the blood helps to decide if a myocardial infarction has occurred.

Defibrillation. The delivery of electric shock to the heart to revert a life-threatening cardiac arrhythmia.

Diastolic. One of the two blood pressure measurements normally taken. It represents the blood pressure in the arteries during the period when the heart is filling.

Dysrhythmias. See *Arrhythmias.*

Echocardiogram. A painless diagnostic test that helps to measure heart function (see *Appendix E*).

Electrocardiogram (EKG or ECG). A painless diagnostic test used to measure the electrical activity of the heart (see *Appendix E*). The commonly used initials *EKG* are derived from the German word for the testing machine used — it was a German invention.

Embolism. A blood clot that forms in the circulation and then breaks loose, traveling through the circulation and eventually lodging in the blood vessels of an organ. Embolism interferes with blood flow to the organ in which it lodges.

Fluoroscope. An x-ray device that enables medical personnel to examine the heart and blood vessels. A fluoroscope is usually used when doctors are trying to position catheters or pacemaker wires in the heart.

Heart attack. Myocardial infarction.

Heart failure. Inadequate pumping of blood by the heart that results in a backup of blood behind the heart. This backup of blood, also called congestion, can produce a number of symptoms: shortness of breath, fatigue, and ankle or leg swelling.

Heart rate. The number of times in a minute that the heart pumps. In other words, the number of heartbeats in a minute. The normal heart rate is between 60 and 100 beats per minute.

Hemoglobin. Oxygen-carrying component in red blood cells.

Holter monitor. A device for following the electrical activity of the heart during a prolonged period of time (usually twelve to twenty-four hours). (See *Appendix E.*)

Hypertension. A condition in which the blood pressure in the cardiovascular system is maintained at too high a level. Long-standing high blood pressure can result in damage to blood vessels in the brain, heart, and kidneys. It is important that patients with hypertension (high blood pressure) receive medication in order to lower their blood pressure to normal levels.

I.V. This abbreviation stands for intravenous. It is the placing of any form of needle or small plastic tube through the skin and into a vein for the purpose of administering fluids or medicines into the body.

Jugular venous pulse tracing. A painless diagnostic test that helps to measure heart function (see *Appendix E, Cardiac Graphics*).

LDH. A chemical substance (enzyme) released from damaged heart cells into the bloodstream. Blood tests demonstrate elevated levels of this enzyme and help in the diagnosis of myocardial infarction.

Monitor. A device used to follow the electrical activity of the heart. This device examines the electrical activity of the heart and determines if abnormal heartbeats (cardiac arrhythmias) are occurring. The electrical activity of the heart is usually displayed on a small television screen. Nurses and physicians working in the coronary care unit frequently watch these screens to see if cardiac arrhythmias are occurring.

Myocardial infarction. Damage to heart muscle that occurs from lack of blood flow in the heart; a heart attack.

Obesity. The condition of being overweight.

Oxygen. A gaseous element essential for life. All the cells of the body require oxygen in order to continue their normal function. The blood carries oxygen to all the cells of the body.

Pacemaker. An electrical device for regulating the heart rate (see *Chapter 8*).

Pericarditis. Inflammation of the membrane that surrounds the heart (see *Chapter 6*).

Pericardium. A tough membrane that surrounds and protects the heart within the body.

Phonocardiogram. A painless diagnostic test that helps to measure heart function (see *Appendix E, Cardiac Graphics*).

Polyunsaturated fat. See *Unsaturated fat.*

Regurgitation. Abnormal backward flow of blood through a heart valve that is not functioning normally.

Saturated fat. A form of fat present in many foods, particularly those of animal origin such as meat, eggs, and whole milk. Diets rich in saturated fat have been implicated as one of the causes of atherosclerosis.

SGOT. A chemical (enzyme) released from damaged heart cells into the blood. Blood tests help to measure elevated levels of SGOT and thereby demonstrate damage to heart cells.

Systolic. One of the two measurements of blood pressure. Systolic blood pressure occurs when the heart is pumping. It is the higher of the two blood pressure measurements.

Tachycardia. An abnormally fast heart rate.

Thrombosis. Formation of a blood clot within a blood vessel.

Triglyceride. A fatty substance found in the blood. Triglycerides are essential to life, but elevated blood levels of these fat substances may contribute to the development of atherosclerosis.

Unsaturated fat. A form of fat commonly found in foods of plant origin such as peanut oil, safflower oil, and corn oil. Eating a diet rich in unsaturated fat does not seem to contribute to the development of atherosclerosis.

Vectorcardiogram. A painless diagnostic test of cardiac electrical activity (see *Appendix E*).

Vein. A blood vessel that carries blood back to the heart. The blood carried in veins has given up its oxygen and is therefore dark in color. Blood in veins also carries waste products away from cells.

Ventricle. The pumping chamber of the heart. There are two ventricles, a right and a left: the right ventricle pumps to the lungs, the left ventricle pumps to the body.

Ventricular fibrillation. Disorganized heartbeat that if not rapidly stopped leads to the death of the patient.

Suggested Reading

A number of writers have vividly described their personal experiences during and following a myocardial infarction and cardiac surgery. These books contain accurate descriptions of the authors' feelings, concerns, and stresses during the period of their illness and recovery. Two of the best accounts are:

1. Halberstam, M., and Lesher, S.: *A Coronary Event.* Philadelphia: J. B. Lippincott, 1976.

2. Nolen, W. A. *Surgeon Under the Knife.* New York: Coward, McCann and Geoghegan, 1976.